Problem-Focused Psychodynamic Psychotherapy

Problem-Focused Psychodynamic Psychotherapy

Fredric N. Busch, M.D.

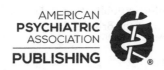

AMERICAN
PSYCHIATRIC
ASSOCIATION
PUBLISHING

If you wish to buy 50 or more copies of the same title, please go to www.appi.org/specialdiscounts for more information.

Copyright © 2022 American Psychiatric Association Publishing

ALL RIGHTS RESERVED

First Edition

Manufactured in the United States of America on acid-free paper
25   24   23   22   21   5   4   3   2   1

American Psychiatric Association Publishing
800 Maine Avenue SW
Suite 900
Washington, DC 20024-2812
www.appi.org

Library of Congress Cataloging-in-Publication Data
Names: Busch, Fredric N., author. | American Psychiatric Association Publishing, issuing body.
Title: Problem-focused psychodynamic psychotherapy / Fredric N. Busch.
Description: First edition. | Washington, DC : American Psychiatric Association Publishing, [2022] | Includes bibliographical references and index.
Identifiers: LCCN 2021021475 (print) | LCCN 2021021476 (ebook) | ISBN 9781615373246 (paperback ; alk. paper) | ISBN 9781615373857 (ebook)
Subjects: MESH: Psychotherapy, Psychodynamic | Psychotherapy, Brief Classification: LCC RC489.P68 (print) | LCC RC489.P68 (ebook) | NLM WM 420.5.P75 | DDC 616.89/147—dc23
LC record available at https://lccn.loc.gov/2021021475
LC ebook record available at https://lccn.loc.gov/2021021476

British Library Cataloguing in Publication Data
A CIP record is available from the British Library.

Contents

About the Author

Dr. Busch is a clinical professor of psychiatry at Weill Cornell Medical College and a faculty member of the Columbia University Center for Psychoanalytic Training and Research. His writing and research have focused on the links between psychoanalysis and psychiatry, including psychodynamic approaches to specific disorders, psychoanalytic research, and psychoanalysis and medication. He has coauthored or authored numerous books on the psychoanalytic approaches to specific disorders, including *Manual of Panic Focused Psychodynamic Psychotherapy*, *Manual of Panic Focused Psychodynamic Psychotherapy—eXtended Range*, *Psychodynamic Treatment of Depression* (now in its second edition), *Psychodynamic Approaches to the Adolescent With Panic Disorder*, *Psychodynamic Approaches to Behavioral Change*, and *Trauma-Focused Psychodynamic Psychotherapy* (in press). Additionally, he is the coauthor of *Psychotherapy and Medication: The Challenge of Integration*. He has been involved in the development of and research on panic focused psychodynamic psychotherapy and more recently on psychodynamic treatment of PTSD.

Acknowledgment

Dr. Busch would like to thank Rosemary Busch Conn, M.D., for her review and suggestions.

Introduction

For many years, and currently in many psychoanalytic institutes, psychoanalysts and psychodynamic psychotherapists have been taught to not be too active, to not focus on symptoms or specific problems, and to avoid psychoeducation. To do so, they're counseled, would disrupt psychoanalytic techniques, including free association and development of the transference, and interfere with the effectiveness of the analytic approach. Over the years many clinicians, particularly those performing psychodynamic psychotherapy, have questioned these shibboleths and encouraged more active approaches in the treatment of patients. The development of symptom- or disorder-focused psychodynamic manuals (see, e.g., Bateman and Fonagy 2016; Busch et al. 2012; Busch et al. 2016; Caligor et al. 2018; Yeomans et al. 2015) provided a basis for the systematic articulation of alternative psychodynamic approaches that incorporated these elements, including more active interventions, a focus on symptoms and associated dynamics, and occasional (although not formal) psychoeducation. In addition, psychodynamic psychotherapeutic manuals required a clarification in terminology and techniques, to make them more user friendly and broadly comprehensible to students and those without psychoanalytic expertise.

I began to engage in the development of panic-focused psychodynamic psychotherapy (PFPP) in 1991 with my colleagues Drs. Barbara Milrod, Theodore Shapiro, and Arnold Cooper (Busch et al. 1991). After training other psychoanalysts in this form of psychotherapy, many of them reported that learning this treatment changed their usual practice. I realized that my own style had changed as well: I was more likely to provide information to patients about how the treatment worked, more focused on specific symptoms, and quicker to suggest a formulation regarding their problems. Although I had concerns about disrupting recommended analytic approaches, I found that patients responded positively to these interventions and rapidly gained an understanding of the process of therapy, how to observe their own intrapsychic states, and how to address symptoms and problems. Subsequent research studies confirmed the efficacy of PFPP for symptoms (Beutel et al. 2013; Milrod et al. 2007, 2016) but also suggested that the impact of focused therapies may be broader, affecting personality issues, behavioral problems, and relationship difficulties. Notably, a recent study (Keefe et al. 2019) found that the focus on specific symptoms and associated dynamics correlated with the effectiveness of treatment in relieving symptoms.

Since the publication of the PFPP manual and the subsequent more comprehensive PFPP, eXtended Range (PFPP-XR) (Busch et al. 2012), there has been extensive further development of symptom-focused psychodynamic psychotherapies (Busch et al., in press). These approaches provide core dynamic formulations for specific disorders along with modified psychodynamic techniques to address particular problems (Table 1). While several different types of disorders have been addressed (depression [Busch et al. 2016], panic/anxiety [Busch et al. 2012], PTSD [Busch et al., in press], personality disorders [Bateman and Fonagy 2016; Caligor et al. 2018; Yeomans et al. 2015], behavioral difficulties [Busch 2018]), there has not been a clear articulation of this overall treatment approach. This book presents such a focused psychodynamic psychotherapeutic approach that can be adapted for patients in general. Rather than one specific aspect of patients' difficulties, problem-focused psychodynamic psychotherapy (PrFPP) focuses on a set of problems (e.g., symptoms, relationship issues, behavioral difficulties). The therapist works with the patient in identifying and addressing the overlapping and unique dynamics of the various problems. This more general approach makes it highly usable for both students and experienced clinicians in addressing a range of patients' difficulties.

This treatment can be employed as a short-term or more extended intervention. Such an approach is of value in that many patients do not want to commit to a longer-term treatment and others lack access to interventions other than brief, focused treatments. With PrFPP, the therapist and patient can rapidly identify, engage, and address core problems and teach self-observational tools that patients can use after treatment.

The book describes how to make a problem list (e.g., symptoms, behavioral issues, relationship difficulties), in part by using psychodynamic exploratory techniques, and examines the context and emotions surrounding each issue. Working with a problem list helps the therapist to maintain a focus despite addressing various difficulties. These initial approaches aid in developing a psychodynamic formulation, providing a framework for identifying and addressing the dynamic contributors to the various problems. The working-through process demonstrates how specific dynamics emerge in different contexts and overlap in contributing to problems. For instance, conflicts about angry feelings viewed as potentially disruptive to close relationships can contribute to both panic symptoms and unassertiveness. These approaches speed the development of patients' self-reflective capacities and the identification of their own dynamics, thus more rapidly addressing core difficulties. The work enables the continued use of modes of managing problems after the treatment is completed.

This book was completed just as the advent of COVID-19 and the subsequent upheaval that it created occurred. People were broadly affected in almost every aspect of their lives. Impacts included anxiety about the virus, isolation through quarantine, conflicts among those quarantined together, disruptions or loss of

TABLE 1. Psychodynamic theory and approaches to specific disorders

Disorder	Psychodynamic theory	Psychodynamic treatment approaches
Panic disorder	Those vulnerable to panic onset have a fearful dependency on others. Anger and autonomy feel threatening to these insecure attachment relationships. Panic displaces these fears in part to the body and provides a means to seek attachment and deny any threat from anger ("I'm helpless and sick. I need you. I'm not a danger").	Focus on the context and feelings surrounding panic episodes to help identify meanings of symptoms. Identify core dynamics: fear of disruption of close relationships, threats from angry feelings, and defenses against anger and separation fears (undoing, reaction formation, denial). Address problems in interpersonal relationships, including fears of assertion and frustration with unresponsive others.
Agoraphobia	Agoraphobic symptoms are attempts—typically unconscious—to manage conflicts surrounding anger, autonomy, and separation, as well as fears of lack of control. Internal conflicts are externalized to dangers in the environment. Patients' fears add to dependency on others and reduce the perceived threat from anger; anger may be expressed indirectly in a coercive effort to control others.	Clarify the content of patients' symptoms to identify and address underlying aggression and separation fears, including in the transference. Explore why patients may avoid exposing themselves to fearful situations as they gain an understanding of symptoms (but there is no formal exposure).
Social anxiety disorder	Underlying feelings of inadequacy and fears of rejection by others can trigger compensatory grandiose fantasies. Conflicted wishes to exhibit oneself and outshine others are associated with unacceptable aggression, triggering guilt and self-punishment.	Identify the context, fantasies, and emotions surrounding experiences of social anxiety. Explore and address feelings of inadequacy, conflicted aggression, and guilt-ridden grandiose and exhibitionistic fantasies. Identify these dynamics as they emerge in patients' overly critical view of themselves and expectation of others' negative judgment.

TABLE 1. Psychodynamic theory and approaches to specific disorders *(continued)*

Disorder	Psychodynamic theory	Psychodynamic treatment approaches
Generalized anxiety disorder	Fears of usually unconscious conflicted feelings and fantasies becoming out of control create the need to maintain constant vigilance, with worries displaced to the body or other areas of patients' lives (e.g., finances, external environment).	Identify conflicts regarding aggressive, sexual, and dependent wishes, which patients fear will be out of control. Recognize the role of hypervigilance as an effort to manage these wishes. Identify how fears of the external environment or the body are displaced from intrapsychic fears.
Posttraumatic stress disorder	Overwhelming trauma triggers dissociation, rage, fear of loss, and unconscious repetition of trauma. Rage at perpetrators can lead to identification with the aggressor, which triggers intense guilt.	Identify the function, meaning, and impact of dissociation. Explore conflicted feelings brought on by trauma that fuel dissociation and other symptoms. Identify sources of guilt that trigger self-punishment, such as identification with the aggressor and survivor guilt. Focus on factors, such as an effort to control trauma, that lead to reenactments.
Cluster C personality disorders (i.e., avoidant, dependent, obsessive-compulsive)	Conflicts about aggression and dependency wishes fuel chronic passivity, avoidance, inhibition of autonomy, and angry feelings characteristic of these disorders.	Identify and address conflicted aggression to detoxify it, leading to improved ability to assert oneself, increased autonomous function, and less need of support from others. Interpret passivity, aggression, and dependency in the transference to facilitate these shifts.
Major depression	Narcissistic vulnerability (sensitivity to rejection) fuels conflicted aggression, as well as compensatory high self-expectations and idealization of others, triggering recurrent disappointment. Conflicted aggression leads to guilt, self-criticism, and depressive symptoms.	Identify and address conflicted aggression to detoxify it, easing guilt. Provide recognition of overly high expectations of self and others to help avert disappointment, anger, and low self-esteem.

TABLE 1. Psychodynamic theory and approaches to specific disorders *(continued)*

Disorder	Psychodynamic theory	Psychodynamic treatment approaches
Borderline personality disorder	Inability to modulate and tolerate negative affects, such as rage or envy, leads to fears of destroying a needed "good" other (Kernberg 1967). A split perception of others as "all good" or "all bad" defensively focuses rage on the devalued bad other, protecting idealized attachment figures. Splitting interferes with the development of more complex views of self and others and a more consolidated identity, adding to dysregulation of negative emotions. Disruptions in mentalization capacities interfere with patients' ability to accurately identify motives and emotions in self and others.	Address intense rageful feelings and fantasies, along with split and shifting self and other representations as they emerge with the therapist, to help clarify and manage the intolerable feelings and defensive splitting (Yeomans et al. 2015). Work to develop patients' mentalization capacities (Bateman and Fonagy 2016).
Narcissistic personality disorder	Patients' underlying low self-esteem, often suppressed, triggers compensatory idealized views of themselves and others who recognize their specialness. These idealized expectations lead to recurrent disappointment with others' actual responses. A reactive rage and devaluation of others who criticize them or do not recognize their specialness develop. Frequent anger, disappointment, and limited empathy toward others disrupt close relationships.	Explore the circumstances in which patients feel disappointed and enraged at others for not adequately recognizing their capabilities or responding to their demands. Identify feelings of inadequacy and efforts to manage self-esteem through idealized self-views and expectations of others. Inevitable disappointment and rage at the therapist provides the opportunity to identify and ameliorate these dynamics in the transference.

Source. Adapted from Busch et al. 2012.

work, and social and political upheaval. In addition, there was a shift in how therapy was performed toward almost entirely remote work. PrFPP is particularly well suited to dealing with these difficulties, as problems can be addressed as they preceded, were affected by, or emerged with the impact of the virus.

As noted above, prior books on focused psychodynamic psychotherapies have been limited to addressing specific subpopulations rather than a treatment that can be used for most patients. After reading *Problem-Focused Psychodynamic Psychotherapy*, clinicians can consult texts on specific disorders for more details on treatments of these particular problems (Bateman and Fonagy 2016; Busch 2018; Busch et al. 2012, 2016, in press; Caligor et al. 2018; Yeomans et al. 2015). As with other books of this nature, there will be many case examples, and psychodynamic factors and techniques will be described in experience-near and relatively jargon-free terms.

References

Bateman A, Fonagy P: Mentalization-Based Treatment for Personality Disorders. New York, Oxford University Press, 2016

Beutel ME, Scheurich V, Knebel A, et al: Implementing panic-focused psychodynamic psychotherapy into clinical practice. Can J Psychiatry 58(6):326–334, 2013 23768260

Busch FN: Psychodynamic Approaches to Behavioral Change. Washington, DC, American Psychiatric Association Publishing, 2018

Busch FN, Cooper AM, Klerman GL, et al: Neurophysiological, cognitive-behavioral and psychoanalytic approaches to panic disorder: toward an integration. Psychoanal Inq 11:316–332, 1991

Busch FN, Milrod BL, Singer M, Aronson A: Panic-Focused Psychodynamic Psychotherapy, eXtended Range. New York, Routledge, 2012

Busch FN, Rudden MG, Shapiro T: Psychodynamic Treatment of Depression, 2nd Edition. Washington, DC, American Psychiatric Publishing, 2016

Busch FN, Milrod BL, Chen CK, Singer M: Trauma-Focused Psychodynamic Psychotherapy. New York, Oxford University Press (in press)

Caligor E, Kernberg OF, Clarking JF, Yeomans FE: Psychodynamic Therapy for Personality Pathology: Treating Self and Interpersonal Functioning. Washington, DC, American Psychiatric Association Publishing, 2018

Keefe JR, Solomonov N, Derubeis RJ, et al: Focus is key: panic-focused interpretations are associated with symptomatic improvement in panic-focused psychodynamic psychotherapy. Psychother Res 29(8):1033–1044, 2019 29667870

Kernberg O: Borderline personality organization. J Am Psychoanal Assoc 15(3):641–685, 1967 4861171

Milrod B, Leon AC, Busch F, et al: A randomized controlled clinical trial of psychoanalytic psychotherapy for panic disorder. Am J Psychiatry 164(2):265–272, 2007 17267789

Milrod B, Chambless DL, Gallop R, et al: Psychotherapies for panic disorder: a tale of two sites. J Clin Psychiatry 77(7):927–935, 2016 27464313

Yeomans FE, Clarkin JF, Kernberg OF: Transference-Focused Psychotherapy for Borderline Personality Disorder: A Clinical Guide. Washington, DC, American Psychiatric Publishing, 2015

1

Developing a Problem List

In this chapter I will describe how the therapist and patient create a list of problems to be pursued in problem-focused psychodynamic psychotherapy (PrFPP) and how this effort aids in establishing the psychotherapeutic process. The therapist helps the patient to clarify difficulties that have not been fully defined and to address barriers to recognizing problems (e.g., denial, shame). The therapist works with the patient to develop self-reflective capacities and understand that problems have meanings and functions. Specific problems then become a lens through which contributory dynamic factors are formulated and addressed. Rather than viewing a problem list as static, the therapist uses psychodynamic techniques to further elaborate and clarify the nature of specific problems over time, as well as identify previously unrecognized difficulties when they emerge in treatment. In addition to defining areas of focus for psychotherapeutic intervention, this process enables work on the therapeutic alliance by allowing therapist and patient to collaborate on the goals of treatment, including resolution of problems.

Identification of Problems

Understanding the Types of Problems

Problem areas can roughly be divided into symptoms/disorders, personality factors, behavioral issues, and relationship difficulties (Table 1–1). This categorization mirrors the series of focused psychodynamic psychotherapeutic ap-

---

TABLE 1–1.   Initial phase of PrFPP: identifying problems

Types of problems

  Symptoms

  Personality factors

  Relationship difficulties

  Behavioral issues

Recognizing the problem as a psychological issue

Defining the extent and impact of the problem

---

proaches, including those for depression (Busch et al. 2016), anxiety (Busch et al. 2012), and PTSD (Busch et al., in press); personality pathology (Bateman and Fonagy 2016; Caligor et al. 2018; Yeomans et al. 2015); and behavioral change (Busch 2018). In general, psychodynamic treatment manuals have not targeted interpersonal difficulties (see Caligor et al. 2018 for an exception), although such difficulties have been addressed as they related to the dynamics of the central problem; relationship issues are an important focus of PrFPP.

Therapists and patients should consider each of these categories in elaborating a problem list, but because there can be significant overlap, the boundaries between these problem areas are fluid. For example, unassertiveness can be viewed as a combination of symptom, personality, behavioral, and relationship difficulties. Problem areas, however, do not have to be clearly categorized for the therapy to proceed effectively; **the language and components of problems will be defined by the therapist and patient as they elaborate their understanding of and approaches to areas of difficulty**. For some patients, it can be helpful for the therapist to develop a shorthand term that can be used to allude to specific problems, such as "your anxiety," "your struggle with low self-esteem," "your communication problems with your spouse," or "your difficulty managing your temper."

Clarifying the Nature of the Problem and Its Psychological Basis

Some problems are readily identified by patients, whereas others are not for a variety of reasons (Table 1–2). Some difficulties are experienced as a natural part of the patient's self or life, or can occur reflexively, almost out of the patient's awareness. In these instances, the therapist works with the patient to recognize the problems as such, indicating that something can be done to relieve or improve them. For other problems there is an active resistance to acknowledging them, consciously or unconsciously (see section "Barriers to Addressing Problems"

TABLE 1–2.	Initial phase of PrFPP: addressing barriers to identifying problems

Denial

Guilt and shame

Intrapsychic conflict and defense

Examples

    Impulse-control problems

    Personality disorders

below). In these cases, the therapist uses psychodynamic approaches to help the patient identify the difficulty and understand the source of the patient's struggle. It is not unusual for problems to be unrecognized due to both a lack of recognition and an unconscious resistance.

Case Example

Ms. A, a 24-year-old woman, presented for treatment of severe anxiety. In the course of the evaluation, the patient alluded to struggles with motivation, but did not discuss them further. The therapist returned to this topic later in the interview:

> THERAPIST: So tell me more about your problem with motivation.
> Ms. A: I'm not sure if it's relevant. I'm really here for my anxiety, but okay…I get very excited and involved in a project. Then as it's nearing completion, I totally lose interest. Not just in that project; in all of my work. I just kind of stall out and don't do anything sometimes for a couple months, until a new project comes along.
> THERAPIST: What causes you to lose interest?
> Ms. A: I don't know. I've never really thought about it. It goes all the way back to grade school. I'm like really moving along with something and then boom, no interest.
> THERAPIST: Well, I think there's something important to understand about what triggers these episodes.
> Ms. A: Why?
> THERAPIST: I think by understanding more about it we could help you to address the problem. And maybe it's even related to your anxiety.
> Ms. A: I've never really considered that anything could be done about it. I thought it's just how I operate. That would be interesting to think about why it happens.

On the basis of this pattern, the therapist also considered and explored the possibility of attention-deficit disorder. Over time, it emerged that the patient associated effective motivation with aggression and was conflicted about it as well as anxious. She felt most threatened when a project was moving toward completion. Recognition of the emotional basis of this problem, once the problem was identified, aided in its relief over time, as well as provided additional information about what was making the patient anxious.

Other problems are not recognized as psychological or emotional difficulties because they are believed to be due to something wrong with the body. For instance, patients with panic disorder are often convinced that certain symptoms are of somatic origin and are surprised to learn after thorough evaluation that nothing is medically amiss. The therapist provides psychoeducation that, because a medical basis for these symptoms has been ruled out, the source is likely psychological and emotional, and patients would benefit from therapeutic work to identify these factors. Somatization often functions as a defense against conflicted feelings and fantasies through a displacement to the body.

Defining the Extent and Impact of the Problem

Problems may more readily emerge as the therapist explores the pattern of their occurrence and repercussions. For instance, a patient may report significant anxiety, but the extent and impact of the anxiety (e.g., phobias; inhibitions) on the patient's life may not be evident. For example, a patient presenting with panic attacks (readily identified as such) became aware in the course of the initial psychiatric evaluation that she struggled with intense anxiety and unassertiveness in a number of areas of her life (at work, in close relationships):

Case Example

Ms. B, a 25-year-old nurse, experienced the onset of panic attacks a few days after a patient of hers died suddenly. She did not know the patient particularly well but viewed the death as "unfair," because the patient was young and much improved. As the period preceding panic onset was explored, she described intense anxiety in two important areas of her life. She felt "underpaid and overworked" in her job and would become fearful and frustrated when feeling under pressure to fulfill her hospital duties, and highly anxious in her relationship with her "cold and callous" boyfriend.

> THERAPIST: Tell me more about how you felt with your boyfriend.
> Ms. B: It was like he gave 10% and I gave 110%. Every time I was with him, I would get really anxious.
> THERAPIST: This was before you had the panic attacks?
> Ms. B: Yes.
> THERAPIST: What were you worried about?
> Ms. B: I was frightened that he was going to break up with me. Looking back, I'm not sure why I stayed with him so long. I was so frustrated inside.

THERAPIST: Did you say anything to him about your frustration?

Ms. B: I didn't want to be a complainer. My dad always told me I was one, and I didn't want my boyfriend to think of me in that way.

THERAPIST: What did you think would happen if you did complain to your boyfriend?

Ms. B: I don't know. That would be pretty scary. I would explode maybe. And I'm sure he would have gotten furious. Maybe the whole relationship would end. But I guess that happened anyway.

This early exploration demonstrated that Ms. B experienced significant anxiety in several areas of her life preceding the onset of panic. In addition, the evaluation revealed one of the dynamic factors in her anxiety: She had difficulty acknowledging her frustration, and when she expressed angry feelings, she would become frightened. She would tend to take back her angry comments. For example, after expressing vengeful fantasies toward her boyfriend, she said, "But I'm not a grudgeful person." Her comments suggested that she feared her anger would disrupt her relationships, indicating separation fears common in panic patients (Busch et al. 2012). History taking further revealed many years of hypochondriacal symptoms and an anxious childhood with a temperamental father and fearful mother. As the evaluation proceeded, Ms. B acknowledged: "I guess I'm just an anxious person. I didn't realize how much it affected my life."

Case Example of an Initial Assessment in PrFPP

The following case provides an overview of identifying a problem list and obtaining information about contributors in the early phase of treatment.

Ms. C, a 46-year-old married woman working in public relations, presented with a primary complaint of anxious and depressed mood, including decreased motivation and interest, reduced appetite, and decreased concentration. She also described social anxiety, and fears of confrontation. The treating therapist concluded that she met criteria for generalized anxiety disorder along with some depressive symptoms and would benefit from a trial of escitalopram. On the baisis of the stressors described below, the therapist told her that psychological and emotional factors contributed to these symptoms and recommended weekly psychodynamic psychotherapy.

The therapist proceeded with exploring the onset of the depressive and anxious symptoms to identify contributors to these problems. Therapist and patient determined they occurred in the context of two stressors that had been developing over the preceding several months. One problem involved the patient's daughter, Heather, the youngest of two children, who was in her senior year of high school and was applying for college. Ms. C reported that she and Heather had always been "very close," and she was feeling upended by **intense**

sadness about her daughter leaving home. In exploring the history of this problem, the therapist learned that the patient had significant difficulty with Heather's aging over many years. She was very attached to the time period before Heather was 10, when Ms. C returned to work and felt sad about the loss of childhood activities they did together. Indeed, Heather never attended camp or sleepovers and spent much of her time, well into adolescence, at home rather than going out with friends. Ms. C's older son, Brian, had a more typical level of involvement outside the home and spent much more time away from the family. He occasionally expressed frustration at the amount of time his mother spent with his sister and sometimes complained that Heather was her favorite.

Her relationship with Heather had intensified when Heather was age 5 during a period in which Ms. C's husband, an entrepreneur, was working particularly hard and often not home at night. She described Jim at that time as not only very busy but increasingly irritable and critical as he became more successful in his work. Subsequently however, Jim suffered setbacks in his business. He worked very little at the time when Ms. C presented, although he was always considering new projects, and she earned the bulk of the family money at her public relations job.

The therapist began an initial exploration into the problems with her daughter:

Ms. C: With her going off to college I feel so sad, and I'm worried it will get worse.

THERAPIST: What do you anticipate it will feel like?

Ms. C: I'm worried about feeling lonely or empty. I mean Brian's around, but Jim and I are pretty distant. I also regret not having a third child. Jim really objected, and I didn't want to create trouble with him.

THERAPIST: What problems would that have caused?

Ms. C: Well, he was really irritable at that time because he felt so stressed about his job. He would just end up attacking me, saying that neither of us had time for another kid, and why didn't I focus on taking on more of the chores in the home first or go back to work? I'm fearful of confrontation and don't push for what I want. So after he yelled at me, I just withdrew from the discussion. I essentially gave up.

THERAPIST: What frightens you about confrontation?

Ms. C: I worry it's going to create a rift. It's certainly like that with my father. I get angry at his criticisms but I'm hesitant to say anything to him. And I guess it's true about with my boss as well.

THERAPIST: So maybe it's a pattern?

Ms. C: Yeah, I guess I never really like confrontation.

As seen in this exchange, Ms. C's **problems with assertiveness** began to emerge in the context of elaborating her separation fears from her daughter and became more apparent in exploring a second major source of distress, **frustration with her work**. The patient described a history of feeling unappreciated at her job at the PR firm. Although she did well and was considered highly successful by her peers, she believed she was underpaid, especially when she learned in recent months that others at her level received a higher salary. Nev-

TABLE 1–3. Problem list for Ms. C
1. Anxious and depressive symptoms
2. Intense sadness about her daughter going to college
3. Difficulties with assertiveness
4. Frustration with her work and boss
5. Feelings of inadequacy and low self-esteem
6. Social anxiety
7. Marital tensions

ertheless, she was fearful of addressing this problem with her boss, a man who had been an important mentor to her for many years. In spite of generally feeling unappreciated, she had always felt recognized by the boss as his "right hand woman" and had some satisfaction from this perception.

About two years prior to presentation, a younger man, Ajay, joined their group. The boss seemed quite taken by him and had been giving him increasing responsibility. Ms. C believed that he had limited talent for the job, and that her boss was blinded by his being a man, his youth, and his social skills. She felt frustrated and also became concerned that Ajay was being relatively well paid and might soon have a salary that approximated hers. She obsessed over whether to talk to her boss about the problem with her salary and the limitations of her coworker but was deeply hesitant to confront him. She believed that in spite of their long history of a good relationship, she could not predict how he might respond if she confronted him about these issues. She also feared that because she was a woman, her boss would react more negatively to her asking for a raise that he would a man. As her frustration persisted, she began to feel less enthusiastic about her work and put less effort into it.

In the context of exploring her problems at home and work, Ms. C reported long-standing **feelings of inadequacy**. She felt embarrassed about the college she had attended, believing that it was not prestigious and that her father was disappointed in her for going there. She believed that others would not respect her PR job because her firm was not as well known as some companies. She was **anxious at social gatherings**, fearing others would look down on her, and had few close friends. She also felt uncomfortable with her husband's friends, believing them to be more high-powered and successful. These feelings combined with her sense of regret about certain decisions she made and with her fears about asserting herself. Finally, Ms. C experienced ongoing **marital tensions** and felt unable to communicate with her husband. Based on this information the therapist and patient identified an initial problem list (Table 1–3).

Additional aspects of how the therapist and patient addressed these problems will be described subsequently.

Barriers to Addressing Problems

As noted above, with many problems the patient may demonstrate an inability or aversion to acknowledging or designating them. Understanding these interfering factors is important for both identifying problems and areas of distress or intense negative feelings (see Table 1–2). Some of the more prevalent obstacles are denial, shame and guilt, and intrapsychic conflicts and defenses. Although these factors interfere with a range of problems, prominent examples include substance use and other impulse-control problems, about which the individual is often in denial or deeply ashamed; personality disorders, in which the patient views the issue as part of who he or she is; and some interpersonal problems, in which the patient does not want to recognize his or her own contribution to the difficulties. Cultural factors can also play a role, because some subgroups react to psychiatric problems with shame or denial. The therapist works with the patient to identify painful feelings and defenses (Freud 1936) that interfere with problem recognition.

Denial

Denial functions as a defense mechanism in which the individual repudiates or will not acknowledge the reality of his or her internal state (e.g., feelings or fantasies) or external reality (illness, climate change, the impact of COVID-19). Denial is a common reaction to painful aspects of reality and can be adaptive in coping with difficult circumstances. However, areas in which a patient rigidly holds on to magical thinking may create significant danger or damage. Denial is commonly associated with substance abuse problems but can be found with a broad range of difficulties. The therapist works to tactfully address the patient's denial and identify what makes the problem painful or frightening to accept:

Case Example

THERAPIST: Tell me about your pattern of drinking.

MR. D: I don't really think there's any particular trigger. Certain days I just start drinking. I could drink like 10 to 12 beers. But it's not really a problem for me. I can handle that much.

THERAPIST: Well, it seems like a lot. When did you last drink?

MR. D: Two days ago.

THERAPIST: So tell me about what happened that day.

MR. D: I felt frustrated about my work. I got into a really bad mood and decided to just put it away for a while. When I got home, my girlfriend was like "What's wrong?" I told her and she said: "Well, you can't just not do the work." I was furious. Of course I know that. I just kind of stomped off and started drinking.

THERAPIST: That sounds like a very specific precipitant.

MR. D: Yeah, it does. It usually doesn't work like that.

THERAPIST: Well, we should look at some other examples to see if that's the case. Did you talk to her about your frustrations?

> Mr. D: No...what's the point? It doesn't get anywhere.
> Therapist: We might want to explore other ways of dealing with these tensions with her.
> Mr. D: Okay. But I don't think the alcohol is a problem. Most days I don't drink.
> Therapist: But when you do is it usually that many drinks?
> Mr. D: Yeah, I guess so.
> Therapist: I think you might have trouble acknowledging your drinking is a problem.
> Mr. D: Well, my Dad was an alcoholic. I don't drink like he did.
> Therapist: Maybe that's part of why it's hard for you to acknowledge the problem, because you don't want to be linked to him. I'm not saying you're an alcoholic, but it sounds like you do have a problem with drinking,
> Mr. D: Yeah, well if I do have an issue it's nothing like he had.

The therapist may note to patients that denial is a common part of substance use problems and disorders and that being able to more consistently recognize and control the use of substances will be part of treatment.

Guilt and Shame

Guilt and shame are common symptoms but also can interfere with identification of other problems. Thus, patients may be embarrassed to reveal certain aspects of their difficulties, including thoughts, feelings, and experiences that they are ashamed of, behaviors that they are critical of, or traumatic events for which they partly blame themselves. The therapist works to identify the presence of shame and guilt as well as the way these feelings block identification of other problems. One example is obsessive-compulsive disorder, in which patients may feel ashamed about the degree of their symptoms, such as handwashing or checking, and tend to minimize or dismiss them. The therapist's nonjudgmental stance aids in the emergence of various issues in the course of treatment. Therapists may reassure patients that their concerns or symptoms are common and explore what is making them anxious or guilty about revealing their difficulties.

If patients demur from revealing a problem (stating, for example, "I don't feel comfortable discussing that"), the therapist can suggest that it would be helpful to explore their concerns and hopefully over time they can feel safe enough to describe them. Many patients take several sessions (or sometimes months) to reveal something that they feel particularly ashamed about, such as a history of abuse or troubling sexual fantasies. In other instances, patients are unconscious of what is causing guilt and shame, and therapists need to address the conflicts and defenses that are interfering with awareness of these feelings (see next section).

Ms. C made a reference to "sometimes having attitudes and behaviors that are like my father," whom she was very critical of. The therapist made an effort to learn more about these:

THERAPIST: Can you tell more about these attitudes?

Ms. C (*appearing uncomfortable*): I don't like to say too much about them.

THERAPIST: I have some ideas about what might make that difficult for you, but can you describe what's making you uncomfortable?

Ms. C: You know I feel very critical of him, so it's kind of embarrassing that I behave like that. Like I'm so mad that he's so controlling, but I can be like that too.

THERAPIST: Well, it's good you're able to recognize that. It's actually not an unusual pattern. Can you give an example?

Ms. C: Yes. If the family is doing an activity and I don't want to do it, I just kind of pout. I'm obviously not having fun.

THERAPIST: Is this like what your father does?

Ms. C: Well not exactly. He decides what he's going to do, and he just does it no matter what anyone else says.

THERAPIST: I see. So he won't even try to participate.

Ms. C: Yes, but I still see myself as being similar. Even though it's not quite the same. And I really don't like to talk about it, although I know we probably should.

THERAPIST: I suspect those difficulties have been hard to address because you keep them cordoned off even from yourself. If we learn more about them I think it will help you to manage these feelings and behaviors better. And we have to understand more about why you equate yourself to your father, when you at least have some perspective on your behavior.

Intrapsychic Conflict and Defense

Intrapsychic conflicts (Freud 1926/1959) and defenses (Freud 1936), while important to elaborate in any psychodynamic psychotherapy, represent other sources of difficulty in identifying problems. Patients may struggle, consciously or unconsciously, with accessing aggressive, dependent, or sexual wishes that trigger anxiety or guilt, which will be elucidated over the course of a successful treatment. For example, a patient's conflict about aggressive feelings and fantasies, associated with fears of disrupting important relationships, can lead to minimizing tensions and submissive behavior with a partner or spouse. Ms. C (see below), for example, took several sessions to acknowledge the extent of her problems with her husband, based in part on fears of her anger.

Problems in Which Barriers to Acknowledgment Are Common: Some Examples

Impulse-Control Problems

Problems controlling impulses can occur in a variety of forms, including temperamental outbursts, poor control of sexual urges, and various forms of addictive behavior (American Psychiatric Association 2013). Patients may deny these types of difficulties, which are sometimes brought to their attention by others. Alternatively, patients may experience painful feelings, such as guilt and shame, in the context of having thought about or acted on these impulses. For example, they may enact sexual behaviors in response to strong sexual urges or a wish for intimacy, but regret doing so with someone unlikely to be a long-term partner or outside their primary relationship. Or they may buy items when in debt, or excessively use drugs or alcohol, followed by intense self-criticism. More severe forms of these impulse-control disorders can require specialized treatment interventions, such as addiction specialists, rehab, or a form of anonymous meetings. Psychodynamic psychotherapeutic approaches targeting problems, however, can often be of value in modulating these difficult to control impulses, especially in less severe forms. Identifying the context, feelings, and fantasies along with contributory dynamics can provide additional tools in regulating these urges and behaviors. In addition to Mr. D whose case was described earlier, many examples of dealing with these problems will be described in this book.

Personality Problems

Personality problems are a source of persistent difficulty for many individuals that are important to define and address. Patients with personality disorders typically do not recognize these attitudes and behaviors as problems, seeing them as part of who they are, creating inherent barriers to acknowledging them. Additionally, patients can feel injured or threatened by designating a problem as part of their personality, and suggesting the patient has a personality disorder may exacerbate this reaction. Furthermore, patients can demonstrate certain features of a personality disorder (American Psychiatric Association 2013), but not others, or have issues or behaviors that meet some of the criteria for different personality disorders, complicating referencing a problem as a specific personality disorder. Therefore, with personality issues, the therapist should work to identify the specific characteristics as part of the problem list in ways that are acceptable and comprehensible for patients. For example, problems with assertiveness, difficulties controlling impulses, and being avoidant of others are terms that may help patients to define and acknowledge these issues.

Narcissistic traits represent a particularly sensitive area for patients, because they are likely to view pointing out these characteristics as attacks and be dismissive or angry in response. Such problems may be more acceptable when described as sensitivity to rejection or low self-esteem (see Chapter 7). Once these concepts are introduced, other narcissistic issues may, over time, be identified as reactions to these vulnerabilities. Thus, the therapist can suggest that a patient's sense of certainty or pressure to be "special" may represent an attempt to compensate for feelings of inadequacy. One patient, for example, was outraged when a close friend told him he suffered from narcissistic personality disorder, and he demanded to know if the therapist corroborated this diagnosis. The therapist stated that rather than trying to determine whether someone met criteria for the disorder, he found it more useful to explore whether a patient suffered from self-esteem issues and problems associated with them, such as being very reactive to slights. The patient was willing to consider this sensitivity as one of his problems, as he often felt criticized by others, although he blamed it primarily on others' lack of recognition of his talents.

Interpersonal Issues

In the case of interpersonal conflicts, patients may describe certain difficulties with others but not recognize the role they play. They may find it upsetting to consider their contribution, wanting to believe the fault lies entirely with the other person. In these instances, the therapist works to tactfully address patients' difficulty identifying these problems, often involving recognizing parts of themselves or behaviors that are painful to acknowledge.

Ongoing Emergence and Clarification of Problems

In PrFPP problem lists are not considered to be static. As sessions proceed, there is both a clarification of problems already being explored and an identification of new problems. New problems can emerge through further exploration of the patient's mental life and environment and identification of blocks that are inhibiting addressing problems (denial, guilt, intrapsychic conflicts, and defense) as described earlier. In the following example, the degree of Ms. C's problems in the relationship with her husband emerged through additional exploration. It also became clear that she had been reluctant to discuss these difficulties.

In a subsequent session Ms. C began to talk about her marital problems in greater depth. It emerged that she was uncomfortable discussing her long-term frustrations with her husband. She described him as driven and perfectionistic, with a very clear idea about the right way to do things. He was often critical of Ms. C's cooking, even though she was working more hours than he was. Although he had been irritable in the past from increased work, he was now frustrated about the setbacks in his entrepreneurial efforts. He would snap at her to "mind her own business" or "fuck off" if she tried to ask questions about his work ventures.

> THERAPIST: So how are you affected by his temper?
> Ms. C: I guess I get kind of quiet and I eventually apologize, even though I don't think I should.
> THERAPIST: How do you end up doing that?
> Ms. C: Well, the whole thing is really painful. In some ways it's easier to talk about separating from my daughter.
> THERAPIST: This situation with your husband seems quite relevant to that. Because when your daughter is gone, you're going to be alone a lot more with him. In fact, this may be significantly adding to your worries.
> Ms. C: That makes sense. I mean I love him, but he can be very difficult. And often I just feel alone when I'm with him.

TABLE 1–4.   Initial phase of PrFPP: therapeutic interventions

Identifying problems

Developing self-reflective skills

Establishing that problems have meanings and functions

Enhancing the therapeutic alliance

Identifying relevant dynamics

Recognizing and exploring the impact of cultural factors

Combining psychotherapy and medication

Other Early Therapeutic Interventions

In addition to identifying the nature of the patients' problems, as discussed earlier in this chapter, other therapeutic tasks are important in paving the way for an effective treatment (Table 1–4). These include developing self-reflective skills; establishing meaning and symbolization; enhancing the therapeutic alliance; identifying relevant dynamics; recognizing and exploring the impact of cultural factors; and combining psychotherapy and medication. The ways in which PrFPP can be useful in enhancing these interventions are described.

Developing Self-Reflective Skills

Assessing the nature of patients' problems aids in the development of their self-reflective skills. The therapist encourages patients to attend to their own thoughts, feelings, and motivations and to explore triggers and contexts of the onset of problems and their persistence. The therapist helps patients recognize that emotions and contexts surrounding problems provide intervention points for addressing and relieving them. As they improve at these tasks, patients learn that problems are more discrete as opposed to an amorphous source of distress. They come to see problems as distinct rather than as an inherent part of themselves or caused by others, thereby creating the potential to relieve them. In addition, patients gain a better sense of control by identifying contributors and triggers of problems.

Establishing That Problems Have Meanings and Functions

In identifying and designating problems, the therapist communicates that they have particular meanings and functions for patients, which are often maladaptive.

Thus, defining problems and early exploration of context and feelings are methods for establishing symbolization. For example, the therapist clarifies that somatic symptoms have a psychological and emotional basis, and therefore have a meaning for the patient. Focus on the body can represent poorly symbolized emotions, a defense against painful feelings and fantasies, or a symbolized representation of an intrapsychic conflict, often involving dependency or aggression. In designating the somatic states as a symptom, the therapist suggests that understanding their meanings and function will contribute to relief. The process of designating symptoms, behaviors, and relationship difficulties as meaningful problems is a core part of this therapy.

Enhancing the Therapeutic Alliance

Working to identify the nature of specific problems enhances the therapeutic alliance (Greenson 1965; Horvath et al. 2011), because the therapist directly addresses what is distressing the patient. In elaborating the context and history of problems, the alliance is further established as the patient begins to recognize the value of these interventions and collaborate with the therapist in this effort. The therapeutic relationship can be used as a model for working together and communicating with others in addressing problems. Interpretations of the transference (Cooper 1987) (see Chapter 2) help the patient understand various reactions to the therapist and become aware of inhibitions and conflicts that interfere with relationships. Disruptions in the relationship with the therapist are key moments to explore, as they can help identify areas of vulnerability that create difficulties in extratherapeutic relationships.

Recognizing Relevant Dynamics

Defining underlying dynamics that are contributory to various problems is a key aspect of this therapy. Often preliminary dynamic information can be identified in creating a problem list. In an early session, for example, a therapist may note that the patient tends to take back his or her comments or feel guilty after expressing anger. In the case of Ms. C, conflicts about angry feelings and fantasies toward others, in which she feared potential damage or disruption to relationships, began to emerge as a factor in several problem areas, including her avoidance of discussing difficulties with her husband. Over the course of the treatment the therapist explored this dynamic's contribution to various symptoms (anxiety or panic, depression), personality difficulties (unassertiveness), relationship issues (failure to express needs and dissatisfaction in relationships), and behavioral problems (e.g., passive aggressive behaviors, as anger could not be expressed directly).

Recognizing and Exploring the Impact of Cultural Factors

Recognizing and exploring the impact of cultural factors is a key area of consideration in the identification and treatment of problems. Patients' cultural backgrounds strongly influence both the nature and perception of their difficulties and what problems they feel safe or unsafe discussing. Some subcultures are more likely to experience certain forms of trauma, such as through the impact of institutionalized racism. Patients may not feel understood unless such factors are taken into account, interfering with the alliance and their comfort in revealing problems. Ms. B, for example, described the influence of her Catholic background on her perception of her revenge fantasies:

> Ms. B: I'm a Catholic, and I learned that if you try to hurt someone, you're going to get it right back. You'll be punished.
> THERAPIST: But you actually haven't acted on these fantasies. Is thinking the same as doing?
> Ms. B: Well no. But I believe I shouldn't even be having these thoughts.
> THERAPIST: I think it's important to explore these fears further and obviously your religion has a big impact on how you feel about these things.
> Ms. B: Yeah, I thought these ideas didn't affect me so much anymore, but maybe my schooling had more of an effect than I realize.

Combining PrFPP and Medication

Much has been written about combining medication with psychotherapy in the treatment of various symptoms and disorders. In PrFPP, medications are used as another method for relieving problems (Busch and Sandberg 2007). While recognizing anxious or depressive disorders as physiologically based and treatable with medication, this approach also views environmental and psychological factors as contributory and symptoms as having important meanings and functions. This model can be conceptualized with the metaphor of a river with physiological, environmental, and psychological/emotional tributaries flowing into it. Overflow of the river represents the anxious or depressive disorder. In any given instance, the degree of contribution of the different components (tributaries) varies. Therefore, addressing physiological, environmental, and psychological/emotional factors can aid in providing relief of symptoms and problems. Difficulties with medication will not be a focus of this book but may become an issue in treatments in which they are used. For example, patients may struggle with shame about needing medication or noncompliance. Psychodynamic understanding can often be of help in addressing issues that arise with medication.

References

American Psychiatric Association: Diagnostic and Statistical Manual of Mental Disorders, 5th Edition. Arlington, VA, American Psychiatric Association, 2013

Bateman A, Fonagy P: Mentalization-Based Treatment for Personality Disorders. New York, Oxford University Press, 2016

Busch FN: Psychodynamic Approaches to Behavioral Change. Washington, DC, American Psychiatric Association Publishing, 2018

Busch FN, Sandberg L: Psychotherapy and Medication: The Challenge of Integration. Hillsdale, NJ, Analytic Press, 2007

Busch FN, Milrod BL, Singer M, Aronson A: Panic-Focused Psychodynamic Psychotherapy, eXtended Range. New York, Routledge, 2012

Busch FN, Rudden MG, Shapiro T: Psychodynamic Treatment of Depression, 2nd Edition. Washington, DC, American Psychiatric Publishing, 2016

Busch FN, Milrod BL, Chen CK, Singer M: Trauma-Focused Psychodynamic Psychotherapy. New York, Oxford University Press (in press)

Caligor E, Kernberg OF, Clarkin JF, Yeomans FE: Psychodynamic Therapy for Personality Pathology: Treating Self and Interpersonal Functioning. Washington, DC, American Psychiatric Association Publishing, 2018

Cooper AM: Changes in psychoanalytic ideas: transference interpretation. J Am Psychoanal Assoc 35(1):77–98, 1987 3584822

Freud A: The Ego and the Mechanisms of Defense. New York, International Universities Press, 1936

Freud S: Inhibitions, symptoms and anxiety (1926), in The Standard Edition of the Complete Psychological Works of Sigmund Freud, Vol XX. Translated by Strachey J. London, Hogarth, 1959, pp 75–175

Greenson RR: The working alliance and the transference neurosis. Psychoanal Q 34:155–181, 1965 14302976

Horvath AO, Del Re AC, Flückiger C, Symonds D: Alliance in individual psychotherapy. Psychotherapy (Chic) 48(1):9–16, 2011 21401269

Yeomans FE, Clarkin JF, Kernberg OF: Transference-Focused Psychotherapy for Borderline Personality Disorder: A Clinical Guide. Washington, DC, American Psychiatric Publishing, 2015

2

Using Psychodynamic Techniques

This chapter will outline how psychodynamic techniques can be oriented toward addressing specific problem areas (Table 2–1). These approaches include development of self-observational skills, linking, free association, clarification and confrontation, interpretation, working with transference, working with dreams, working through, and working with countertransference. The use of genetic (developmental), defense, and transference interpretations in relation to specific problems will be described.

Development of Self-Observational Skills

Self-observation, a component of mentalization (Fonagy and Target 1997), is a critical process in examining factors contributing to problems. Patients enter treatment with varying capacities for self-observation; the therapist plays an essential role in teaching and enhancing this ability. This effort begins at the start of treatment in identifying problems and continues in exploring the surrounding context, mental states, and emotions. The therapist works with the patient in obtaining an expanding picture of what occurred prior to the development of problems and attending to triggers of fluctuations in severity. A diary for mon-

17

TABLE 2–1.   Psychodynamic techniques in addressing problems
Development of self-observational skills (reflective capacity)
Linking
Free association
Clarification and confrontation
Interpretation
Working with transference
Working with dreams
Working through
Working with countertransference

itoring context, thoughts, and feelings surrounding problems can also promote the use of this skill (Busch 2018).

Metaphors can be useful ways to communicate about the process of self-observation and examine triggers relevant to problems. One way of describing the monitoring of intrapsychic states, environmental stressors, and behavioral patterns is the notion of building a scaffold. Just as a scaffold allows closer and safer observation of and access to a structure that needs repair, self-observation enables the identification of problems and their sources. The elaboration of context and a psychodynamic formulation provide a series of intervention points for relieving problem areas (see Chapter 4). Another way of describing this stance is comparing it to reviewing a videotape of certain problems to see how one is feeling and reacting to the relevant circumstances. New strategies can be derived and tested on the basis of these analyses. Both metaphors emphasize the concept of stepping back and evaluating with the observing ego.

Another metaphor that can be useful in developing self-observational capacities is viewing problems as "whirlpools." The notion of a whirlpool can capture a patient's sense of spinning, lack of control, and being trapped by problems. In an analogy as to how patients may have difficulties recognizing a problematic state, the therapist can compare how one cannot see a whirlpool when one is pulled down into it. Key steps include identifying that the patient is in a whirlpool and understanding the nature of it (e.g., anxiety, panic attacks, depression, personality problems, and relationship difficulties). The therapist can then discuss what landmarks (e.g., context, emotions) signal the location and nature of the whirlpool. Once the whirlpool is recognized, the patient can work on ways to get out. In the analogy, the patient can strengthen her swimming muscles, or get a float (e.g., medication), or get another person (the therapist) with a boat to help her.

Once the patient is out of the whirlpool, it is important to identify currents that tend to draw the patient back toward it. These currents can include particular self and other representations, intrapsychic conflicts, relationship patterns, and impulse-control difficulties. One might say to the patient: "Once you are aware of these currents you can work to steer yourself to calmer waters, away from being dragged toward the whirlpool."

Case Example

Ms. E, a 32-year-old single woman, became caught in catastrophic anxious thoughts about being permanently alone when she was having problems with her boyfriend, who had been married previously:

> Ms. E: I get caught in my negative emotions. I feel furious and rejected that my boyfriend won't commit to our relationship. I feel there's no one else out there for me.
>
> Therapist: It sounds as if you feel there's no possible positive outcome for you. It's as if you're caught in a whirlpool that makes it impossible for you to look at this problem and realize there are alternative ways you might handle it.
>
> Ms. E: Yes, that's exactly right. I can't see things clearly. I feel there's something terribly wrong with me that he's rejecting me for.
>
> Therapist: I know you've mentioned before that he has a very tough time committing to anything. You said he even backs out of seeing his own children.
>
> Ms. E: That's true. He always has one foot out the door. But I do feel there will be no one else for me.
>
> Therapist: And at other times you've mentioned there are other men interested in you. When you're not in the whirlpool, you think and feel very differently about the situation. I think we need to understand what triggers your being in this state.
>
> Ms. E: It's when I'm trying to reach him, and he doesn't even answer my texts. Sometimes for a full day! But then he always gets back to me. But during that time I think, "This is it. It's all over."
>
> Therapist: I guess one thing we need to consider is why you stay involved with somebody who behaves like this. And then we want to understand why his not returning your text feels so catastrophic! Especially when you say he always eventually gets back to you. One thing that comes to mind is how abandoned you felt by your father. You said he was away for months, and you weren't sure where he was.
>
> Ms. E: Yeah, and my mom just looked sad. We never talked about it though.
>
> Therapist: Well, I think this is one current that pulls you toward the whirlpool. It's important to understand how you were affected by your father's absences and why you have trouble confronting your boyfriend when these feelings come up.

Therapists and patients should also be on the alert for factors that can disrupt self-observation, just as they work to identify emotions, memories, and defenses that interfere with recognizing problems (see Chapter 1). These elements can include shame, anxiety, conflicts, or trauma linked to what the patient is addressing at that time. Certain psychologically or emotionally based bodily states can elude self-observation because they have not been symbolized in psychological terms and are viewed as something wrong with the body. For instance, somatic sensations indicative of anxiety and rage may not be recognized as such and potentially trigger catastrophic worries (e.g., palpitations as a heart attack). Therapists can call attention to a sudden interruption in self-observation as an indicator of emotions or conflicts that should be explored.

Linking

This therapeutic intervention identifies how patients' problems are linked to particular aspects of their emotions, stressors, fantasies, self and other representations, and their history. Linking also plays a role in making bodily experiences meaningful by connecting sensations and perceptions with particular intrapsychic and environmental contexts. This gives the patient an opportunity to understand how their problems have developed and further establishes their meaning. For example, in the case of Ms. B (see Chapter 1), her panic attacks were linked to frustrations with her work and former boyfriend, fears of expressing her anger, and a developmental history of family conflict involving an anxious mother and temperamental father.

The concept of these factors being unlinked or problematically linked can be useful in identifying the impact and manifestations of adverse or traumatic events. Trauma can interfere with the linkage between bodily information and memories of the trauma (dissociation), increasing the likelihood somatic states will be experienced as medically dangerous and not symbolically meaningful; this disconnection increases the potential for developing catastrophic cognitions, somatic symptoms, panic attacks, phobias, and acting-out behaviors. For instance, a veteran may experience intense chest pain and fear in response to feeling threatened by someone on the street but may not link this to terrifying confrontations with enemy combatants on the battlefield. Additionally, intrapsychic conflicts between wishes and internalized prohibitions can lead to a defensive delinking in an attempt to reduce unbearable conflicts or emotions. Thus, individuals with panic may repress angry feelings when they feel others are not responding to them, causing them to focus on unrelated catastrophic fears.

Trauma triggers intense negative emotions and can also lead to inaccurate linkages to sensations directly associated with the traumatic experience, such as particular sights, sounds, and smells, triggering fear or panic. Problematic linkages can occur between perceptions of traumatic events with internal fantasies and cognitions (e.g., I was irresponsible or selfish; therefore, this trauma happened to me). In these instances the therapist works with the patient to 1) recognize these links, which may be unconscious, and 2) separate the connection between particular sensations and fantasies from the past trauma that is causing them to be viewed as dangerous. For instance, the therapist would work with a veteran to recognize that loud sounds heard on the street are not indicative of being attacked by an enemy.

Free Association

In the technique of free association the therapist encourages the patient to say whatever comes to mind. The technique is meant to help the patient avoid screening specific thoughts, feelings, and fantasies, allowing the therapist access to mental states that feel conflicted and trigger emotional discomfort. Inherently, patients will suppress certain mental states in spite of this approach, and the therapist should be alert to the patient's hesitation or avoidance of particular mental contents. In problem-focused psychodynamic psychotherapy, the therapist will work with the patient's free associations to make clarifications and interpretations targeting problems. This approach is used, for example, in helping patients to identify contributory feelings and fantasies.

The therapist, for example, encouraged associations to get further information about Ms. C's (see Chapter 1) inability to ask her boss for a raise:

THERAPIST: What comes to mind about asking the boss for more money?

Ms. C: I don't know. He's actually a nice guy, so I don't know why I would be worried. But then again, when it comes to talking about money, I've seen him get kind of stern. So I guess he could get angry about a raise request. (*Patient pauses for a moment.*) I'm embarrassed to say this bothers me, but now he likes Ajay so much. And I think I've told you I was his "right hand woman." So it just seems to me that maybe he doesn't even favor me anymore, and that may be confirmed if I make the request. I'll be displaced.

THERAPIST: I think it would be good to understand why you're uncomfortable revealing that it upsets you that the boss favors Ajay. But what comes to mind about being displaced?

Ms. C: I think of my brother. Somehow my father always just seemed to connect better with him. He didn't get the same criticism I did. And just because he was good at sports. Even though my Dad claimed academics was most important, he didn't really act like that.

THERAPIST: So maybe this helps to understand another aspect of why you feel so threatened about asking the boss. You're overly worried about being displaced by your co-worker, like with your brother. And also we know you're angry about Ajay. Maybe that's giving you trouble.

Ms. C: I guess I'm angry. I know I've kind of lost motivation at work. And I do think it's unfair that the boss thinks he's so great when he's really not.

In this instance allowing the patient to freely associate helped to link her current worries with childhood fears about being displaced by her brother. As described previously, the therapist and Ms. C had made a connection between her fears and her father's judgmental attitude toward her. In dealing with problems there is typically more than one dynamic factor that contributes, and addressing these various factors can be important for improvement. The patient was very uncomfortable about discussing her feelings about her brother, likely related to conflicts about her anger and jealousy. The free-associative process, and the therapist's nonjudgmental stance, helped the patient acknowledge these painful memories of displacement. The process also sharpened the patient's self-observational skills by learning how following her thoughts helped identify an important contributor to her unassertiveness.

Clarification and Confrontation

Clarification and confrontation are techniques in which the therapist points out a patient's typical patterns of thought, feelings, or behavior (Stone 1981). They are used to bring attention to problematic cognitive, emotional, and behavioral patterns or a characteristic mode of perception that adds to the patient's difficulties. Confrontation identifies a pattern of contradictory sets of beliefs, attitudes, or actions that the patient appears to be unaware of. These techniques aid in the development of the patient's capacity for self-observation by distinguishing patterns in his or her mental life and behavior.

Clarification and confrontation are also used in identifying problems, along with particular affects, fantasies, or conflicts that act as triggers or contributors. Examples might include: "I notice that when you become frustrated with your wife, you withdraw and avoid her rather than address the problem you are having with her." Or "I've observed that when you feel threatened at work, you attack one of your subordinates rather than acknowledge the uncomfortable feelings you are having."

Case Example

A confrontation is illustrated in the following exchange with Mr. F, a 54-year-old man who struggled with motivational problems and passive aggression:

> MR. F: I can't understand how I end up with others being angry with me. I can't deal with their anger. It's the last thing I want.
> THERAPIST: You say that you don't want to have tensions with others, and yet you often feel rebellious and procrastinate when other people ask you to do tasks.
> MR. F: I guess it's true. I really don't think about what I might have done to trigger their anger.
> THERAPIST: We should try to understand why you don't think about it. When you feel pressed to do something you don't want to do you

really get furious. You don't believe that you should have to complete these tasks, like washing the dishes.

MR. F: When I'm mad and refusing to do things, I don't really care about
the impact it may have on others, like them becoming angry.
Even though if I thought about it I would know my wife will be
mad that the dishes are stacking up. But I don't see any solution to
this.

THERAPIST: I think we need to explore how this split takes place and
help you to realize that when you're rebelling others are likely to
get mad. Maybe at that point you can think, "I don't want to do
this task, but I know the other person will get angry if I don't. So
maybe it's better for me to push ahead and do it."

Interpretation

Interpretations link observed emotions, thoughts, and behaviors to the dynamic factors that contribute to them. The therapist suggests how specific, typically unconscious, intrapsychic conflicts and defenses contribute to problems
and may connect these factors to the transference and the patient's history. Interpretations are developed and modified over the course of treatment, providing a growing framework of dynamic factors and interventions relevant to
problematic symptoms and behaviors. They are elaborated in different contexts
in the process of working through, a phase of therapy in which dynamics are explored in greater depth and a variety of approaches to problems are investigated
(see below and Chapter 9).

There are various subtypes of interpretations, including those focusing on
conflicts, defenses, developmental factors, and the transference. A conflict interpretation describes an often-unconscious wish or fantasy and the internalized prohibitions and emotional reactions that it triggers, such as guilt or fear.
A common example would be identifying a wish to harm another person, leading to anxiety and guilt about damage to others and fears of retaliation. Therapists may also interpret two wishes that are experienced as contradictory, such
as to be close to and hurt another person.

Defense interpretations consider the ways in which patients characteristically defend themselves from painful affects, negative perceptions of themselves and others, or threatening unconscious fantasies (see Chapter 4). These
defenses typically operate outside of awareness, and patients' learning about
how the defenses affect them is important for addressing problems. For example in the defense of identification with the aggressor (Freud 1936), individuals
link their self-image with someone whom they experienced or fantasized as
having power and dominance, particularly someone with whom they were vulnerable in the past. Patients may unconsciously use this defense mechanism to
combat feelings of inadequacy and gain a sense of being empowered and in control. However, this stance often causes guilty feelings, particularly about wishes
to dominate, hurt, or get revenge on others in ways that had previously made

them feel bullied or threatened. This defense mechanism often interferes with assertive behaviors, as patients can confuse normal assertiveness with wishes and actions that they perceive as damaging.

Case Example

Mr. G, a 52-year-old lawyer with chronic depression, had significant difficulty getting his staff members to complete their tasks properly, because he wanted to be seen as a friend rather than a boss. He accepted weak excuses for their need to leave early or take days off and tolerated shoddy work. However, he would obsess angrily about his employees not adequately doing their job and blamed them in part for the limited success of his practice. Occasionally he would mildly reproach one of them, but this did little to get them to follow his rules.

> THERAPIST: Why do you think you have difficulty making more demands on your employees?
>
> MR. G: Well, I'm scared they'll quit, and then I'll be stuck training a new person. I also want to be seen as the good guy. I don't want to hurt their feelings.
>
> THERAPIST: What do you mean by that?
>
> MR. G: I feel that if I criticize them, I'll get really nasty or abusive and just make them feel very badly.
>
> THERAPIST: I think it's important for us to understand more about this, especially as you don't give any indication you would actually behave that way.

Mr. G's background proved relevant to this issue, as he described his parents as unfair and rigid about rules. He was often upbraided about minor infractions (coming home a few minutes late for curfew) or for not making better grades, even though he found school difficult. He was furious with his parents, but if he got angry directly, his mother would "withdraw her love" and not speak to him for days. This caused him great anguish, and he struggled between his wish to be a "good boy" and his anger at what he regarded as unfair treatment. The therapist discussed with Mr. G how viewing himself as an assertive boss was linked in his mind with his parents' attacks on him, an example of identification with the aggressor.

> THERAPIST: It's interesting that when you describe what you're worried you would do as a boss critiquing your employees, your behavior sounds just like your parents with you.
>
> MR. G: Yes. I guess it does. I mean, I don't want to be unfair and to hurt people the way they did with me. I know what it feels like.
>
> THERAPIST: It sounds as if you really feel guilty when you need to critique your employees, even though you actually tend to be overly polite.
>
> MR. G: Yeah. I've always worried that if I really allowed myself more power, I could really hurt others.

THERAPIST: I think we can help you more with this feeling, particularly because it is so inhibiting and your behavior is so clearly at odds with your fears.

Understanding this defense provided relief of some of Mr. G's problems, allowing him to set better limits with his employees. To this end, the therapist had to detoxify the dangers Mr. G associated with being the authority.

Interpretations focusing on developmental factors, which have been termed "genetic" (as in genesis), link past experiences, perceptions, or fantasies with current thoughts or behavior.

Case Example

Ms. H, a 46-year-old entrepreneur, had difficulties setting boundaries with others who were narcissistically preoccupied or self-focused. She described problems that emerged with someone she had previously thought of as a friend.

Ms. H: I really think Nancy is just not that smart, and I don't want to deal with her.

THERAPIST: What is it about her?

Ms. H: Well it seems like in her fight with her boss, she just wants me to agree with her. And I don't think her boss is that bad. She's calling him names and threatening to report him for harassment. If I try to give her any of my perspective, she just gets mad. I mean she doesn't get it. But then I feel guilty when I think or say critical things about her.

THERAPIST: What worries you about criticizing her?

Ms. H: Well, I just think it's mean to say someone is dumb, and I feel like I'm withholding my support. We were pretty close friends. And then I think you'll think negatively of me if I criticize her intelligence. Don't you think that's bad?

THERAPIST: Well I don't see the problem with your having critical feelings about her. But it also seems to be reminiscent of your father. If you didn't agree with him, he would get furious and attack you for not taking his side. We know you felt very angry but ended up feeling guilty and apologizing to him.

Ms. H: Yes, that's true. She is being like my father in this instance. Acting like she's never wrong about anything. And getting mad if I disagree. I guess I'd like to just stop talking to her about this, because it's upsetting and frustrating, but then I just end up listening to her rant.

THERAPIST: It seems you feel guilty about getting angry at her and that causes you to yield to listening to her. You feel stuck like with your father. We're trying to help you be able to set better boundaries. Helping you to better tolerate you anger would make it easier for you to set limits.

Ms. H: Well, it's important to me that you don't think it's mean to set limits.

Working With Transference

In the transference (Freud 1905/1953), the patient experiences emotions and perceptions of prior significant relationships with the therapist, allowing for more direct exploration and identification of fantasies and conflicts. Interpreting the transference enables patients to understand characteristic ways in which they misperceive others, and how these perceptions generalize to other relationships (see Cooper 1987; Westen and Gabbard 2002). The increased awareness of their feelings, conflicts, defenses, and actions obtained via the transference provides valuable information in building a psychodynamic formulation and addressing problems. Emotions and conflicts regarding the therapist can also help to identify specific triggers of problems, such as a patient's feeling injured or becoming angry. The therapist's nonjudgmental stance in response to patients' mental states is crucial in providing a sense of safety for unconscious fantasies to emerge, as patients typically anticipate a rejecting, critical, or intrusive response.

On occasion patients will demonstrate certain problematic behaviors within the treatment, referred to as *enactments*. For instance, passive aggressive enactments include lateness to appointments or payment of bills. Patients may miss or "forget" a session after discussing a difficult topic or avoid raising an issue that they are frustrated about. These enactments provide additional opportunities to examine problems in the context of the transference relationship, with more direct access to triggering cues, feelings, and conflicts. The therapist should be aware, however, that patients may experience examining transference fantasies, feelings, and behaviors as potentially threatening to the therapeutic relationship.

Case Example

Mr. I, a 46-year-old salesman at a tech company, feared expressing his wishes directly in his close relationships and at work but would alternately lose his temper with his wife, children, and colleagues. He was unassertive when he feared rejection and retaliation for expressing his own needs but would become enraged when he felt others were trying to pressure or control him or disregarded him. For example, after obtaining an important new client at work, he was beset by guilt and anxiety, fearing he had hurt and angered his colleagues or would trigger retaliation from his boss. At the same time he felt furious, believing he was not getting enough credit for this achievement. Exploration of his past history revealed Mr. I's experience of a bullying father as a source of his inhibitions, as he demeaned the patient for his efforts at independence from the family, such as requesting to change their usual vacation plans to a different venue. He anticipated his boss and others at work would react like his father, becoming punitive to demonstrate they were in control and could not tolerate someone else having power. The therapist and Mr. I identified that he felt "caught in the trap" with his

father, both enraged and yet fearful of acting any differently, expecting to be un-
heard or attacked. Understanding these factors had aided him in becoming
bolder at work, which helped him to get the new client.

A significant proportion of therapeutic work with Mr. I was accomplished
through interpreting the transference, where he was able to explore these feelings and anticipated dangers in a safe, exploratory environment. Mr. I typically
viewed the therapist as his strict controlling father with whom he also felt
"trapped." He feared that the therapist would reject him if he were to be successful or if he were to complain or argue about what he saw as the "rules" of therapy.
He viewed the therapist's starting and ending the sessions on time and having a
due date for monthly payments as "obsessional" and overly strict. In one session
the patient noted that he had delayed payment of the fee because he was frustrated by so many bills and that he would pay next time. The therapist believed
that it was not productive to set an absolute limit with the patient but did feel his
enactment should be brought into the discussion.

> THERAPIST: That's fine to pay next time, but I think we should note that
> the payment is late and that there's something important about
> doing this with me.

The patient did not respond to this comment but in the next session said:

> MR. I: I was very angry that you said the payment was late.
> THERAPIST: Can you tell me more about those feelings?
> MR. I: I think you just like to be in control of things, and you got mad
> that I was saying I would bring it in next time. I think you were
> saying I was misbehaving.
> THERAPIST: My sense was that you were aware it was late and that's why
> you were telling me you would bring it next time. It seemed im-
> portant to you to feel some control with me so that you could ex-
> press your frustration about the payments. But it sounds like
> somehow you heard my response as a reprimand.
> MR. I: It gave me a sense of freedom in being able to wait to pay you.
> But then it did sound like you were criticizing me.
> THERAPIST: That's when I believe you see me like your father, refusing to ac-
> cept any compromise and criticizing you for disagreeing with him.
> MR. I: That's certainly what it's like, but I do see how this is different.

In a related circumstance the patient brought up how he was angry at the
therapist about the time boundaries of the session, stating that he felt "bottled
up and angry":

> MR. I: I was angry that I didn't get to call my internist before I came here.
> THERAPIST: What were you angry about?
> MR. I: Well, I had it on my list to call him about my lab results, but then
> that would cause me to miss part of the session. So since I'm pay-
> ing for it that could be quite a bit of money.

THERAPIST: So what triggered your anger? It sounds like you thought about it and you made the decision that made the most sense to you.

MR. I: Well, I'm mad that I can't come 5 minutes late and just stay the extra 5 minutes. I don't like that you're in control of the time.

THERAPIST: Yes, I can see that, although it's important for me to keep on schedule. I think you would also be mad if I tended to run late for appointments.

MR. I: I get that, but I don't like it. And I definitely think you could be a little more flexible.

THERAPIST: It sounds like you're viewing me as very rigid and that you feel "caught in the trap," as if I'm your father.

MR. I: He is very rigid. He's like the emperor at home and at his job. And you definitely can't disagree with him. He just gets furious and says, "You should learn your place," even though I'm now a grown man.

THERAPIST: I guess one important difference here is that you're able to express your frustration with me.

MR. I: That's true even though I'm still mad you won't be more flexible. But I don't have that bottled up frustrated feeling anymore. I feel a lot more relaxed.

Working With Dreams

Working with dreams helps the therapist gain information about patients' unconscious wishes and defenses (Altman 1975; Freud 1900/1953). In approaching a dream, the therapist explores associations patients have to the different elements (thoughts, feelings, and images) in the dream. In decoding a dream, the therapist considers the relevant dynamic factors and the state of the transference, as well as thoughts and feelings about current experiences that appear in the dream. The therapist explores what different elements may symbolize for patients through the associative process, rather than imposing preset meanings.

Case Example

Mr. J, a 46-year-old laboratory technician, presented with severe recurrent depression, including suicidal ideation, and vegetative symptoms. His symptoms responded somewhat but not completely to medication, despite trying a broad range of antidepressants and mood stabilizers. During these depressive periods he was intensely self-critical, feeling "stupid" and incompetent. He even blamed himself for not doing a better job at heading off his depression. He feared he would "mess up" projects at work, despite having generally good reviews and excellent attendance, even during his most severe symptoms. His self-attacks would alternate with feelings of rage toward his family.

Mr. J described his mother as intensely critical and otherwise neglectful of him and to some extent his two sisters. He viewed her as very self-involved, focused on her appearance, and dismissive of pressing emotional and physical needs of her children. Mr. J also reported that his mother favored his sisters and that they were often allied against him. Mr. J was closer to his father, who, however, did nothing to prevent the critical attacks of his mother. In addition, his father died when Mr. J was 20 years old. This left him feeling trapped with a critical family and no allies, and with conflicted anger at his father for not supporting and then abandoning him.

Mr. J had been discussing a recent frustrating visit with his family that triggered anxiety, depression, and anger. At that time he reported a dream:

MR. J: My mom was making me do a repetitive task, involving a basket of laundry. I didn't want to do it, and it was making her mad. Mom said, "Linda doesn't mind. She gets all As. She goes to a good college." And I said, "I go to a good college. Williams in Williamstown." My mom replied, "Linda goes to Queens College for free." Then I took a donut that was packed with a grenade and contemplated putting it in my mouth.

In associating to the dream he reported:

MR. J: Well, my Mom was always making me do a lot of chores and is constantly criticizing and insulting me. And Linda was a person I met on a trip. She was a kind of jerk, like she knew everything. For instance, she had kids and said she knew exactly what limits to set with their behavior. Very irritating. I'm not sure what else.

THERAPIST: Well, it seems like Linda is kind of like your sister Susan.

MR. J: That makes a lot of sense. My Mom never criticized her but was always attacking me. Susan's a know it all, as you know. And it's weird because her son did go to Queens College. And Susan got straight A's. It was so unfair that I was criticized all the time, and she didn't get any trouble. My mom was always mean to me.

THERAPIST: What do you think about the donuts?

MR. J: Well, it was weird that it had a grenade in it. Was I about to eat it? Maybe it was triggered because I'm going to visit a relative my Mom doesn't like. And I don't visit my Mom. I know she would be mad.

THERAPIST: But you do answer back to your mom in the dream. It's not like you just accept the criticism. And you stop before eating the donut. I don't know if you're deciding whether to ingest it or throw it at her. Because we know when you internalize your Mom's criticisms, you're viciously self-critical. And you blame yourself. It's like an explosion. But when you are in touch with your rage at her you do better.

MR. J: Yeah. I am having way less of those episodes now. But now I'm mad she's even in my dreams. It's annoying that she's still present.

THERAPIST: But it's better for this to be in your dream than to experience such distress inside when you're awake. And to not eat the donut!

MR. J: That's true.

Mr. J's anger was internalized as he accepted blame and viciously attacked himself. It was if the trauma were recurring directly with his mother but was taking place inside his own mind. His intense self-criticism typically triggered severe depressive symptoms. Interpretations that explained that he was behaving as if the trauma were recurring but that his current reality was much safer helped him recognize the source of his distress. Understanding how he internalized his mother's attacks, directing his anger at his mother toward himself, provided relief for the self-criticism and helped the patient say more directly what was on his mind. The powerful image of the dream of the donut containing a grenade represented the explosive damaging nature of his actual maternal experience, and gave a vivid, concrete, and symbolic understanding of a choice he could make with how to manage his anger.

Working Through

Working through (see Chapter 9) involves the process of identifying various dynamic contributors to symptoms and behavioral issues and understanding how they emerge in different contexts and circumstances. This phase of therapy is important in relieving problems, which tend to persist in part because of the multiple contributing factors and functions that they serve. These dynamics can emerge and affect behavior in a variety of contexts, including with partners, bosses, and friends. Over the course of treatment, the patient develops an increased awareness and understanding of these dynamics, examines them in a variety of circumstances, and is made aware of increased opportunities and strategies to intervene with problems. For instance, patients may need to first become aware of anger that is denied before they can tolerate and accept anger, identify triggers of these feelings, and learn to express anger appropriately. Several examples of working through are provided in the book, including in Chapter 9.

Working With Countertransference

Clinicians should always scan their feelings, fantasies, and responses to patients, as therapists can use this information to avoid enacting problematic countertransference reactions and to identify certain experiences the patient is having. These reactions can be an indication of the presence of significant and meaningful transference. Once clinicians become aware of these feelings, they should carefully evaluate what they are responding to in the patient's verbal and nonverbal behavior. Therapists should consider how their own dynamics may affect the intensity of their reaction or emotional response to a patient's particular issue (Gabbard 1995; Sandler 1976). Countertransference not only can provide additional information about the patients' dynamics but also may indicate what kinds of difficulties they may generate interpersonally. For instance, the therapist felt pulled to enter into power struggles with Mr. I about the boundaries of treatment, which echoed the responses of others in his life. Awareness of this urge both helped the therapist to avoid doing so but also aided him in identifying the patient's provocative way of challenging authority, potentially triggering the attacks he greatly feared. It is generally recommended that dynamic therapists have their own treatment during their training to better understand their intrapsychic conflicts and to identify areas of vulnerability to countertransference.

References

Altman L: The Dream in Psychoanalysis. New York, International Universities Press, 1975

Busch FN: Psychodynamic Approaches to Behavioral Change. Washington, DC, American Psychiatric Association Publishing, 2018

Cooper AM: Changes in psychoanalytic ideas: transference interpretation. J Am Psychoanal Assoc 35(1):77–98, 1987 3584822

Fonagy P, Target M: Attachment and reflective function: their role in self-organization. Dev Psychopathol 9(4):679–700, 1997 9449001

Freud A: The Ego and the Mechanisms of Defense. New York, International Universities Press, 1936

Freud S: Fragment of an analysis of a case of hysteria (1905), in The Standard Edition of the Complete Psychological Works of Sigmund Freud, Vol VII. Translated by Strachey J. London, Hogarth, 1953, pp 3–122

Freud S: The interpretation of dreams (1900), in The Standard Edition of the Complete Psychological Works of Sigmund Freud, Vols IV and V. London, Hogarth, 1953

Gabbard GO: Countertransference: the emerging common ground. Int J Psychoanal 76(Pt 3):475–485, 1995 7558607

Sandler J: Countertransference and role-responsiveness. Int Rev Psychoanal 3:43–47, 1976

Stone L: Notes on the noninterpretive elements in the psychoanalytic situation and process. J Am Psychoanal Assoc 29(1):89–118, 1981 7217609

Westen D, Gabbard GO: Developments in cognitive neuroscience: II. Implications for theories of transference. J Am Psychoanal Assoc 50(1):99–134, 2002 12018876

3

Examining the Context, Emotions, and Developmental History Contributing to Problems

As problems are identified, the therapist works with patients to examine the internal and external context surrounding problems, including emotions, fantasies, and environmental triggers (Table 3–1). This exploration aids in the growth of self-reflective capacities as patients learn to attend to specific aspects of their mental life. In elaborating these factors, patients become aware that problems do not come out of the blue but emerge in particular circumstances and emotional states that can be identified, helping to establish their psychological meanings. Understanding these sources is key to making changes in problems by recognizing where they derive from, what difficulties they create, and what alternative options exist for these thoughts, feelings, and behaviors. In this process the therapist works with patients to identify how symptoms and problems are linked (see Chapter 2) to particular aspects of patients' feelings and fantasies as well as relevant developmental history. In addition, the context is used to help identify psychodynamic factors relevant to particular problems. The elaboration of the context, emotions, meanings, and relevant developmental history begins in the initial evaluation of the patient in conjunction with identifying specific problems and continues as part of the ongoing treatment.

TABLE 3–1.   **Examining the context, emotions, and developmental history contributing to problems**

Identifying the circumstances, feelings, and fantasies surrounding problems

Identifying relevant developmental history and traumatic experiences

Addressing disruptions in the capacity to recognize links

Exploring variability in problems

    Variability in different contexts

    Recurrences or resurgences

Identifying relevant psychodynamic factors

Identifying the Circumstances, Feelings, and Fantasies Surrounding Problems

The therapist works with patients to explore environmental stressors, feelings, and fantasies that are triggers of their problems. Some problems have clear precipitating events and affects, whereas others, particularly those that are more long-standing, may not, but all are likely to be exacerbated by particular circumstances. Patients are frequently not aware of these precipitants, and a detailed examination is needed to identify relevant contexts, emotions, and thoughts. The therapist works to engage the patient's curiosity and collaboration in this search for contributors to problems.

Case Example

Mr. K, a 42-year-old lawyer, described panic attacks that interfered with leaving his apartment and caused him to limit his travel. When asked about his experiences, he reported typical symptoms of panic attacks (shortness of breath, palpitations, tremor, worries he was having a heart attack) along with fears of "feeling trapped." When asked what circumstances triggered these symptoms, he described feeling trapped in elevators, a common source of claustrophobia. With further exploration it emerged that the feelings also occurred when he was traveling on the highway, which led him to limit his travel by car. When asked to describe further what frightened him about these situations, the patient reported that when he felt trapped, he also felt alone. He feared something would happen to him medically, and he would not have access to people he saw as safe, specifically his wife and children.

Additional contributors to his symptoms emerged when Mr. K reported a panic episode at work, noting that he did not feel trapped at that time:

THERAPIST: Can you tell me the circumstances of that attack?

MR. K: Well, I was at a meeting with a partner at my firm. He's a very accomplished guy that I admire, and I wanted to impress him.

THERAPIST: You mean impress him about your work?

MR. K: No. I just wanted to impress him as a person. I wanted him to think highly of me. But then I noticed that I felt anxious and had some palpitations. I also get a tremor when I'm anxious. And I thought "Oh no I'm going to have a panic attack. This will be humiliating."

THERAPIST: What did you feel would be humiliating?

MR. K: Well it's pretty obvious. He would notice that I'm anxious, particularly the tremor. Then he would see me as a weak person. He wouldn't be interested in me anymore.

THERAPIST: I think we need to understand more about this. What is this sense of having to impress people that makes you so anxious? And you also don't consider the possibility that someone could have empathy for your anxiety rather than think you're weak.

MR. K: I hadn't thought about that. But the people in my profession are pretty tough. I don't think he would think too highly of me.

Thus, ongoing exploration of the contexts revealed another specific trigger: that his panic would occur "with people I want to impress," as he feared that others would judge him negatively. In exploring his symptoms, the identification of contexts led to some preliminary understanding of situations and mental states that contributed to his panic and phobias, including fears of aloneness and rejection. Also, it suggested the presence of another problem to address, underlying insecurity and a related sense of low self-esteem.

Identifying Relevant Developmental History and Traumatic Experiences

Developmental History

Contexts and emotions that trigger problems typically derive from particular developmental events. The therapist obtains a history to gain information about patients' backgrounds and to identify factors that contribute to specific problems, including relevant adverse or traumatic experiences. The therapist helps patients to construct a narrative for problems and demarcate their presence and form over time. Patients are often not aware of how certain experiences in their past, including traumatic events, have affected their lives and contributed to their symptoms. Indeed, because of the impact of adverse events or trauma, including dissociation, disrupted symbolization, and avoidance of pain, patients may inadvertently or unconsciously avoid acknowledging the relevance of past events to their current lives. Making patients aware of these connections can reduce the overestimation of the danger and lack of control of current circumstances and problems.

After the therapist identified Mr. K's feelings of aloneness and humiliation surrounding his panic episodes, he explored the patient's background with regard to contributors to these fears. The patient noted that he felt very alone growing up; his family was not very affectionate, and its members "expressed little concern for each other." His mother was more interested in her social activities and "left us alone to fend for ourselves." The patient described his father as a "tough guy" who did not express much emotion and was occasionally highly critical of what he referred to as the patient's "laziness." The lack of empathy, his mother's absence, and his father's criticisms contributed to his sense of aloneness and insecurity.

> THERAPIST: So you've talked about being frightened of being trapped and alone or humiliated in front of others. This does seem relevant to events in your past.
> MR. K: I guess I always felt a pressure to be the tough kid, even though underneath that I was always kind of anxious. I didn't feel good about myself, and I wanted to try to appear strong to others.
> THERAPIST: It seems like you still feel that need with others. Except for certain "safe" people.
> MR. K: Oh yes…I still don't feel that good about myself. I haven't accomplished what I could. I'm unable to maintain the suave demeanor I desire to really impress people. And I feel kind of unrecognized for what I have accomplished.
> THERAPIST: I think we want to talk more about those feelings of insecurity to understand your struggles with panic now, because we see that they are interrelated.

This case of Mr. K demonstrates another aspect of problem-focused psychodynamic psychotherapy that will be elaborated in other chapters: the interconnection of problems on a dynamic basis. As described, Mr. K's insecurity added to the intensification of his anxiety to the level of panic attacks. Therefore, addressing insecurity will aid in the relief of panic in addition to his struggles with self-esteem. Indeed, feelings of inadequacy affected a far broader range of Mr. K's psychology than was evident in its emergence in panic. For example, he frequently felt down about his perceived lack of accomplishment and compared himself unfavorably to others he saw as more powerful and successful.

Adverse Events and Trauma

Many sources of evidence point to the role of trauma in the development of a broad range of symptoms, disorders, problematic behavior, and relationship difficulties (Casey and Strain 2016; Kessler et al. 2010). Although obtaining history in the initial consultation will elicit some episodes of trauma, patients may not reveal other incidents because they are ashamed, do not connect the trauma to their current symptoms, or may have repressed the event(s). Sometimes patients (and therapists) avoid exploring traumatic and painful childhood experiences because of the emotional distress they trigger. Therefore, clinicians should be alert to the potential emergence of further information about trauma and other adverse events in the course of treatment. In addition, in the context of persistent posttraumatic symptoms such as phobias, affective dysregulation, and dissociation, therapists should consider additional exploration of traumatic events.

Case Example

In the review of the precipitants of Mr. J's (see Chapter 2) depressive and anxious symptoms, it emerged that the patient would get much worse after visiting with his family. In particular, he would have a surge in self-criticism while at the same time he became furious with his family's behavior.

> THERAPIST: So, what happened at the family visit?
>
> MR. J: Well, my mother started attacking me again. She asked me if I got promoted at my work. She knows that's a sore point for me, and I haven't been. And my sister is a know it all. She started talking about what I needed to do to get promoted. I didn't know why I thought it would go better with them. I always think that and then the same thing happens. Why do I go there even?
>
> THERAPIST: I think that's a good question to look at. What happened after you left?
>
> MR. J: Well, I started criticizing myself about not being promoted. I was saying "Oh you really screw things up at work. You could be doing a lot better. You shouldn't keep putting off projects." Even though I hardly procrastinate at all.
>
> THERAPIST: Clearly your symptoms worsened after visiting home. We have noticed this pattern before. And it's notable that you began to attack yourself with exactly the same criticisms that your mother and sister had of you.
>
> MR. J: I see what you're saying. But I'm still really mad at myself. Why did I let this happen again?
>
> THERAPIST: This is another example of where you criticize yourself for having problems. You're working the best you can to address them.

In this case, the patient continued to be pulled toward repetition of early traumatic repetitions in his recurrently painful interaction with the family. Exploring why he continued to repeat these experiences was an important part of his treatment.

Addressing Disruptions in the Capacity to Identify Links

Often patients have not recognized the links between their problems, their internal states, and environmental stressors (Busch 2017). This lack of connection may derive from not having considered or examined the context and history of their problems. The therapist works to identify these links and develop patients' skills for doing so. However, these linkages may have never formed, or they may have been dissociated or repressed because of painful affects or conflict, creating an aversion to recognizing these connections. For example, patients may not want to acknowledge the link between a phobic symptom and a traumatic experience because it reminds them consciously of the pain of this event. And yet a recognition of this linkage is of value to patients when they are trying to understand the origin of their fears of the phobic situation that are not appropriate in their current circumstances. The therapist points out when patients will not acknowledge what seems like an evident connection or meaning, working to identify the discomfort these links bring up for them.

Case Example

Mr. L, a 32-year-old man, had difficulty examining his angry outbursts toward his children for not immediately responding when he asked them to stop a particular behavior, such as playing a video game. The therapist worked to psychoeducate the patient, who was presenting for treatment under pressure from his husband, that his expectations of the children were unrealistic, as this lack of response was not unusual for children. Mr. L averred that his temper outbursts were appropriate, and it took some time for him to consider that he was overreacting, in part spurred on by his husband's increasing concern about the impact of his behavior on the children. After that acknowledgment he had difficulty exploring the origins of what could be causing such an intense reaction ("I have no clue. My family was fine."). He had trouble contemplating what was happening inside before these episodes occurred and struggled to change the behavior; he intermittently returned to rationalizing that his temper was justified.

Over several sessions of exploring his background, however, it emerged that he felt intense pressures to be the "perfect child," never creating any trouble for his parents, who struggled to manage their own anxiety and irritability. In fact, his father was quite demanding of the patient in terms of his own behavior, being highly critical of any "infractions" that disturbed his parents, often leading to spanking him with a belt. He stated that his father was calm, though distant, when he behaved properly and did what he was told. His view of himself as the "perfect child" became a compensatory myth justifying his father's attitudes and allowing him to feel better about submitting to pressures. It emerged that the patient was highly self-critical of any struggles he had with getting things done efficiently despite his overall success. In addition, he feared rejection for his interests in men, because his father viewed being gay as a defect. Anything less than what he imagined as being perfect triggered severe self-attacks.

The pressures that he felt from his parents and his need to be "perfect" were so ingrained that he had difficulty stepping back and recognizing his temper and self-criticism were problems. Linking his angry outbursts to presumed "misbehavior," perfectionistic expectations, and representations of himself as messy, bad, and needing to be reprimanded was helpful in gaining recognition of the connections of his problems to the past. Another contributory factor became apparent as the patient's underlying rage toward his parents emerged. His anger had previously felt intolerable and had been self-directed or was dealt with through identification with the aggressor. Unconsciously identifying with his father's stern reprimands of him in his behavior toward his children helped him to feel powerful. Some of his resistance to acknowledging the problem with his temper, in addition to what he learned growing up, was the guilt he felt when he consciously realized he was behaving like his father with his own children. Becoming aware of these factors enabled the patient to grasp the damage his behavior was causing and to make efforts to recognize when his rage was building.

Exploring Variability in Problems
Variability in Different Contexts

The therapist notes the specificity of certain triggers of problems and suggests that these contexts are meaningful and important to further investigate. In addition, therapist and patient identify that these problems do not occur or are less severe in other circumstances (if they are not pervasive). It is of value to explore what makes certain situations safer or more burdened by problems than others. For instance, if the symptoms occur with a friend, spouse, or boss, but not with others, what makes interactions with these individuals a trigger? Such problems may involve fears of intimacy or of authority, or both.

Case Example

A 64-year-old businessman was anxious about expressing his needs or opinions with one particular friend and his wife but was quite direct about his feelings with others:

> Mr. M: In most situations I'm an outspoken person. But with Jim and my wife I can't seem to say anything that might upset them, like when I'm angry about something they did. If I get mad at them they will just pull away and stop talking to me, which is very upsetting.
>
> Therapist: That does sound distressing, although it's important to understand why it's so scary that you can't express your negative feelings toward them. Anything come to mind about what frightens you?
>
> Mr. M (*quiet and thoughtful*): I guess it reminds me of my father. When he didn't like what I was saying he would not talk to me for days, giving me the "cold shoulder." And it feels the same way with my wife and Jim. It's very upsetting when someone ignores you for days.
>
> Therapist: Yes, and we need to think about how you might be able to express your frustrations to them, as otherwise you end up feeling thwarted and anxious. One question is whether you've tried

to talk to them about their withdrawal. I know you've said that with your father there was no way to address this problem because of how he reacted.

MR. M: Well, we could discuss talking with Jim and Debbie about it. It sounds scary.

Recurrences or Resurgences of Problems

The therapist should explore what triggers lead to the recurrence or exacerbation of symptoms or problems. This process aids in further identifying and addressing important contributors.

After having improved in the first several sessions of treatment, Ms. C's (see Chapters 1 and 2) depressive and anxious symptoms increased significantly when her daughter did not get into the college of her choice. When this exacerbation was explored, she revealed that this event mirrored a very painful episode in her own life. Ms. C and her parents had hoped she would attend the prestigious college X; however, Ms. C was rejected. Her daughter was rejected by the same college. Her father made derisive comments about Heather getting her "limited intelligence" from the patient, and she feared he might say something directly to her daughter.

Ms. C: I'm really preoccupied about Heather not getting into X, and I'm still feeling down.

THERAPIST: What's upsetting you about it at this point?

Ms. C: Well, I keep thinking about saying to her: maybe you can go to college Y this year, do well, and you can transfer to X next year. But I know this isn't a good idea. It sounds like I'm being critical like my Dad.

THERAPIST: Why do you think you feel pressed to say it to her?

Ms. C: I feel embarrassed, particularly with the other parents. I worry they might not have heard of Y, or that they will be thinking, "Oh I guess she wasn't smart enough to get into X."

THERAPIST: And this will reflect poorly on you?

Ms. C: Yes, I hate to say it, but when I see them I'm worried they're thinking negatively of me. And I say, "Y is where Heather really wanted to go," and they probably think I'm just saying that because I'm embarrassed that she didn't do better.

Ms. C recalled that her father could have done more to help her get into college X when she was applying. He knew someone from his business who had attended the school and was a significant donor. However, as far as she was aware, her father never spoke to him. In addition, Ms. C believed she was unfairly targeted for punishment with a suspension when she and other students were discovered drinking at a suburban home. She stated that she had only had one drink while others were drunk. She believed her counselor subsequently became halfhearted in his efforts on her behalf, interfering with her acceptance by certain schools, as she did not do as well as expected based on her academic record. Again, she felt her father could have done more to blunt the impact of this accusation and punishment on her application process. Although he did little to aid her efforts, her father was highly critical and disappointed when she did not get into her top choice, making comments such as "Perhaps the family brains did not make it into your generation."

As noted in Chapter 1, impulse-control problems can also be exacerbated by particular triggers. Identifying these triggers can aid in better managing these impulsive behaviors.

Case Example

Mr. N, a 42-year-old man discussed in more detail in Chapter 4, reported that he had a resurgence of his drinking problems and was now very depressed, stating that he was "in a dark place." Mr. N felt "trapped" within his job that he suddenly found meaningless and anxious about financial problems. He described growing up with an emotionally abusive father, whom he lived with as an adolescent after his parents' divorce. He rebelled by acting out in multiple ways, including failing at school and drug use but struggled with his rage toward his father and self-loathing. The therapist explored what might have triggered a resurgence of his alcohol use.

> THERAPIST: So, what was going on just before your drinking?
>
> MR. N: I had just been under a lot of pressure with my presentations and I felt trapped. Also, I felt my work was meaningless. And I'm doing a lot of the work on my own. I feel alone. And I'm doing all this work and not seeing the benefit of it financially. I just needed something to get away from these dark thoughts. But after I started drinking it got worse. I just started brutally attacking myself about what a loser I was.
>
> THERAPIST: I don't think alcohol helps to relieve these problems. It seems to me you feel back in the traumatic situation living with your father. In that situation you did feel trapped, alone, disempowered. You were enraged and rebelled, but this just led to more abusive attacks by your father. At some point you turned the rage against yourself. You hardly recognize that a week ago you were feeling pretty good.
>
> MR. N: I was. I was going to the gym regularly. And now I feel trapped and angry. And the alcohol does feel like an effort to rebel, to get out of this place. But it didn't work very well. Then I get down on myself about the drinking.
>
> THERAPIST: We know that going to the gym is a much more effective way to get out of this negative place. I think if you can recognize you're headed in this whirlpool in your thoughts, then you may be able to choose a different path when you feel this way.
>
> MR. N: I'll try to keep in mind what's happening as I have the urge to drink. I really need to stop.

Identifying Relevant Psychodynamic Factors: Exploration of Context and the Psychodynamic Formulation

Exploring and elaborating on the context of problems helps to identify contributory dynamic factors that become components of a developing psychodynamic formulation. This formulation, as will be described further in Chapter 4, can be used as a roadmap to approach problems and shift patients toward greater cognitive and mental control over their difficulties. For instance, Mr. J identified that his distress would surge with any contact with his family, and that he would quickly switch to self-loathing. As the specific self-criticisms were explored, therapist and patient learned that they mirrored those that his mother tormented him with. The information was used to map a preliminary plan for how to address these factors: working to identify the patient's self-criticisms as unfair and to develop an increased tolerance and/or limit setting with the family. Thus, the therapist helped to bring these factors into awareness and use them to establish a mental model for addressing problems.

The following vignette provides an example of the impact of identification of contexts and the early development of a psychodynamic formulation for understanding and modifying problems.

Case Example

Mr. O, a 68-year-old married business consultant, presented for evaluation of depression and anxiety associated with fears of his business sustaining losses and feelings of being "bad" or a "failure." Despite these fears and self-criticisms, his business was profitable, and he was in a financially sound position. He felt guilty about his ex-wife, having been involved with another woman whom he left her for many years previously. Although his ex-wife had complained little about his being absent much of the time, she became furious when he asked for a divorce, and because of his guilt, he overcompensated her financially in the divorce agreement. He was disappointed with his children's lack of financial success and felt worried and responsible for them should he have to stop his business due to aging. He was preoccupied and fearful about death despite his being in good health. Ultimately it emerged that he thought about death as an abandonment or as a punishment.

Mr. O reported that when he was growing up, his parents viewed him as "bad." However, when his history was reviewed, the patient reported he did not do anything terribly unusual for children and believed his parents' impression of him was unfair. Ultimately, information suggested that his "badness" related to his tendency to push limits (e.g., staying out past curfew; driving the car without permission), which was a later mark of his success in business. Nevertheless, he continued to struggle with feelings of being bad throughout his life. He recalled being very upset with the birth of his brother at age 4 and felt "replaced," believing things were never the same again with his parents. In fact, over the years his brother was viewed as "the good one" and behaved well, in contrast to the patient. He took guilty satisfaction at his success relative to her lack of achievement later in life. He recalled one consistently positive figure in his life, his grandmother, who spoke little English. Although they rarely communicated verbally, the patient believed his grandmother conveyed a positive regard for him.

At age 18 Mr. O's parents forced him to go to military training for a year based on continued concerns about his behavior problems. He was frustrated as he was already working in jobs in his area of interest but managed to tolerate the training. As soon as he finished, he began pursuing business opportunities. His efforts were significantly disrupted when at age 23 he was called up to serve in the army reserves based on his prior training. He was furious toward his parents for having put him in that position and thwarting his career.

Understanding, through treatment, the sources of Mr. O's negative self-view and how they contributed to his catastrophic anxiety about his business and finances helped to relieve his symptoms. In examining the contexts of resurgences of his symptoms, patient and therapist identified that his fears and depressive symptoms were triggered by reminders of past business failures but were exacerbated when he felt rejected or alone. For instance, he was prone to becoming frightened about business matters when his wife went on vacation. Using this information, the therapist suggested a psychodynamic formulation of the patient feeling rejected by his parents for being "bad" and internalizing their negative view of him. He reacted angrily to this perception but directed his anger inward, viewing himself as a failure, to avoid further disruption in the relationship with them.

An example of these precipitants occurred just after the therapist went on vacation, when Mr. O felt like a "failure, bad, I've done something wrong. I'm in trouble and have to get away. I'm frightened about my finances. I'm back in the whirlpool." Therapist and patient had referred to "the whirlpool" as his state of being catastrophically fearful about his business. He was in the middle of a deal in which a client's business was failing, in spite of the patient's best efforts. Exploration revealed he had done nothing wrong in this situation, even though he blamed himself. The business was failing in part because his advice was ignored. And indeed, he would lose only some of the significant amount of money he generated from the consultation.

In exploring how Mr. O slipped again into the whirlpool, several factors came up, including the therapist's recent vacation:

Mr. O: I felt very alone in dealing with this. Of course you were away.
Therapist: Yes, and you tend to equate being alone with feeling you are bad, that you're not supported or you're being punished in some way.
Mr. O: I see what you mean. My parents never really recognized what was going on with me. And they wouldn't talk to me during times when I was being punished. And thinking about it, my partner at work is away and my daughter is leaving for an extended trip.

THERAPIST: So that's a number of reasons that you feel more abandoned than usual.

MR. O: And it's interesting because it brings me back to my first business loss 30 years ago. Seeing this business going down the tubes. And that really was scary. I wasn't sure what I was going to do. I didn't have any money and I was borrowing from others. And I was in really bad shape. I really felt alone a that time. I went to a psychiatrist, and he was worried I was suicidal. But I wasn't suicidal at all. Just in bad shape. But he did make me go on antidepressants, which helped me.

THERAPIST: So that was a real danger, not a whirlpool. And it was a traumatic experience for you that contributes to your fears now. I guess you've always felt alone when you're struggling, as you received little support from your parents.

MR. O: And maybe I was more bothered by your vacation than I thought.

THERAPIST: I think that makes sense. And I know that when you feel left alone by others you get mad. But you haven't always felt safe about feeling or expressing that.

MR. O: I do get mad about being left alone. (*smiling and partly joking*) I hope you had a great time!

Identifying the contexts of the patient's catastrophic fears furthered an understanding of contributing dynamic factors. The therapist worked with the patient's equating separation with rejection and his sense of being bad, which were displaced to anxiety about his finances. This formulation helped Mr. O to recognize that the dangers he experienced derived from emotional rather than realistic factors. Being able to address his fears of abandonment and rejection directly with the therapist further helped relieve his anxieties. The patient's expression of frustration with the therapist's vacation in the form of a joke showed an increased safety with his angry feelings and fantasies.

References

Busch FN: A model for integrating actual neurotic or unrepresented states and symbolized aspects of intrapsychic conflict. Psychoanal Q 86(1):75–108, 2017 28272818

Casey PR, Strain JJ (eds): Trauma and Stressor-Related Disorders. Arlington, VA, American Psychiatric Publishing, 2016

Kessler RC, McLaughlin KA, Green JG, et al: Childhood adversities and adult psychopathology in the WHO World Mental Health Surveys. Br J Psychiatry 197(5):378–385, 2010 21037215

4

Developing a Psychodynamic Formulation

Various elements of a patient's mental life, symptoms, and behavioral difficulties can be organized in what is called a *psychodynamic formulation* (Perry et al. 1987), which specifies and integrates these factors. These factors are derived from different psychoanalytic models of the mind (Auchincloss 2015). Early development and communication of a formulation are key components of many focused psychodynamic psychotherapies. Data obtained by examining emotions and contexts of problems provide information to begin building the formulation. Additional elements of a psychodynamic formulation will be described, including self and other representations, developmental factors, traumatic experiences, intrapsychic conflicts, defense mechanisms, and mentalization capacities (Table 4–1). The therapist communicates to the patient the suggested dynamic factors and their relevance to various problems, creating a framework for understanding and addressing them. The formulation is collaboratively added to and adjusted over the course of treatment, further articulating specific emotional and psychological meanings of problems and enhancing the specificity of interventions.

Self and Other Representations

During development and subsequently, individuals form internalized representations of themselves and others that are derived particularly from significant attachment relationships (Bowlby 1973; Freud 1905/1953; Jacobson 1964). These models include perceptions of self and others, as well as the self in interaction with others, consisting of a particular view of the self, an accompanying emotional state, and an expectation of response from others. Individuals have a variety of these representations, although certain forms tend to predominate or lead to problems. These perceptions of self and others exert ongoing conscious and unconscious influences that affect symptoms, conflicts, defenses, personality factors, and relationships. For example, patients with panic disorder frequently view themselves as unsafe, requiring others for protection, and often perceive others as temperamental, controlling, or rejecting, aggravating their sense of insecurity (Busch et al. 2012). Their perceptions add to a sense of fearful dependency on significant others. Alternatively, they may perceive themselves as rageful and others as easily damaged, heightening their fears of anger disrupting important attachment relationships.

Therapists help illuminate the nature of these representations so patients can more objectively examine their influence and formulate approaches to the problems they contribute to. For example, panic patients often have limited awareness of their insecurity with others, and fears of damaging others with their anger are predominantly unconscious. Therapists can identify how these self and other representations lead patients to overestimate the sense of threat with others, when in many instances there is little realistic danger. Therapists can also address the rigidity and extent to which patients tend to hold on to certain representations. As will be discussed in Chapter 8, self and other representations may also be dissociated from one another, leading to a variety of problems. In addition, patients may be in conflict about particular self-representations, for instance when viewing themselves as wishing harm or revenge on others. Therapists can point out how certain perceptions are inconsistent, in conflict, or unintegrated, such as panic patients' feeling threatened by others and simultaneously fearing damaging others. Therapists also work to enhance mentalization skills so patients can recognize that others may be influenced by factors unrelated to patients' expectations.

The supportive, nonjudgmental stance of therapists can aid patients in internalizing more positive models of interactions that challenge the negative ones they anticipate. For example, the therapist's tolerance and exploration of patients' angry feelings and fantasies emphasize models in which the feelings and expression of anger are safer and less damaging.

Developmental Factors

Core aspects of self and other representations are formed in the context of early attachment relationships. According to Bowlby (1973), and ultimately corroborated by observational and epidemiological evidence, insecure and unstable relationships with caregivers, or rejecting and critical behavior, lead to the devel-

TABLE 4–1. Psychodynamic factors that contribute to problems

Self and other representations

Developmental factors

Traumatic experiences

Intrapsychic conflicts

Defenses

Mentalization deficits

opment of negative internal models, such as of the self as inadequate and unlovable and others as unresponsive and punitive. These representations contribute to a vulnerability to psychopathology later in life, particularly in the setting of loss or adversity. Systematic studies of perceptions of parents in patients with anxiety disorders and depression indicate that these patients perceive their parents as rejecting, critical, or lacking emotional warmth (Parker 1983; Perris et al. 1986; Silove 1986). Although current symptomatology may influence such perceptions, they tend to be stable even after resolution of depression or anxiety disorders (Gerlsma et al. 1993; Nitta et al. 2008).

In obtaining the patient's developmental history, therapists explore the family circumstances and history, perceptions of salient relationships (e.g., parents, caregivers, grandparents), relationships among family members, social and intimate relationships outside the family, and cultural factors. Therapists inquire about significant losses, deaths, and separations occurring during childhood and patient and family reactions to them. Adverse and traumatic events, such as severe family conflict, physical or sexual abuse, poverty, negligence, and violence within their community, are explored. Elaborating these developmental factors aids patients in recognizing what contributed to troubling self and other representations, conflicts, and defenses. In problem-focused psychodynamic psychotherapy (PrFPP), therapists work to identify how these developmental factors are relevant and contributory to specific problems.

The following cases demonstrate the development and use of the psychodynamic formulation.

Case Example

Mr. P, a 52-year-old lawyer, presented with fears of traveling in trains and driving his car. He had experienced panic attacks under these circumstances, and his anxiety led him to revise his travel schedule and location where he lived to avoid these situations (Table 4–2). Upon further evaluation it emerged that Mr. P felt considerable anxiety socially and at work, fearing he would be judged or criticized for being ineffective. These worries were accompanied by the sense that he was being pressured by others to perform. Stomach pains would typically occur

---

TABLE 4–2.   Mr. P's problems

---

1. Panic attacks

2. Phobias of driving, trains

3. Social anxiety

4. Somatic symptoms

---

with his anxiety, and it emerged subsequently that he feared losing control and vomiting, which he would find terribly humiliating.

He noted that he avoided others for fear of being reprimanded by them for something inexplicable (Table 4–3) and to avoid being a "burden." He worried about disrupting the relationship with his boss, with a fear of being fired, and that his financial security would be threatened. He had increased anxiety with his wife when she became more irritable after their second child left for college, leaving an empty nest. At the same time that he felt insecure, he had fantasies of being the lead partner at the firm, in charge and in control of others. He felt safe with others who had a calm tone or he felt sure would not attack him.

In exploring his background, the patient reported that his parents fought chronically, eventually divorcing when he was 11. He then lived primarily with his mother, and while his father lived in relative comfort, they struggled to make ends meet. His mother remarried when he was 16, but he despised his stepfather, whom he saw as inadequate, partly because he was unable to keep a job. He described the relationship with his father as alternating between vicious criticisms and neglect. When his father did occasionally visit him at his mother's home, he would walk in unexpectedly and criticize the patient saying, "What are you doing you idiot! You should be working!" He chronically worried his father would catch him lying on the couch and attack him for being lazy, even though his visits were infrequent. His father even lambasted him for playing a game that involved learning strategies, which Mr. P believed nurtured the development of his academic skills. He also worried about being financially dependent on his father, believing that if he expressed too much irritation his father would lose his temper and withdraw support. His father was otherwise preoccupied with his business and was involved in a series of relationships with women. Mr. P's only persistently positive relationships growing up were with a close friend and his friend's family, whom he considered more "normal."

Mr. P reported that he began to rebel in junior high and high school by smoking pot, growing his hair long, and playing in a band. His efforts in school diminished and his grades were average, despite recognizing he could perform better. Mr. P knew that his father would yell at him occasionally about these behaviors, but his father was increasingly absent. Looking back, he saw it as a way of expressing his anger and attempting to engage his father's attention in a provocative manner. However, he also felt badly about "screwing up" in school. Additionally, he felt insecure and socially anxious in groups and with girls, heightening his feelings of inadequacy.

Mr. P's current fears paralleled his experience of attacks by his father. He expected to be viewed as lazy and ineffective and was worried that his boss would

TABLE 4–3.	Mr. P's self and other representations/developmental history

Self and other representations

Self as inadequate or ineffective; others as critical, judgmental, and intrusive

Self as angry, rebellious; others as attacking or easily damaged

Developmental history

Parental conflict and the subsequent divorce disrupted the patient's sense of security. He experienced his father as intrusive and judgmental, alternating with being neglectful. He viewed his mother as being ineffective at helping him and chose a problematic partner.

walk into the room and criticize him just as his father had. He feared being intruded upon or pressured by others, including demands made by his boss and his wife. These feelings persisted despite a recent promotion at the firm. At the same time he muted his anger at others out of a fear he would be attacked and criticized for expressing it. Indeed, he would become anxious in situations where he felt frustrated with others, such as his coworkers, and feared losing his temper.

Case Example

Ms. Q, a 47-year-old female artist, presented with intense feelings of failure, inadequacy, and self-criticism, as well as anger toward her husband and sister for their lack of responsiveness and judgmental attitudes toward her (Table 4–4). For example, she struggled with her anger at her sister after feeling criticized by her at a recent family get together. She had expressed an opinion about a particular college his son was considering, to which her sister replied, "Well I don't think you're an expert about education." She felt stung by this slight but did not express her outrage. Instead, she became very self-attacking about being "so sensitive," identifying her anger at her as wrong and inappropriate and an illustration of her incapacity. She viewed several aspects of her life through the lens of her presumptive failure. For example, despite prior gallery shows and sales of her artwork, her fear of failure hindered her pursuit of painting.

Ms. Q also described significant struggles with her husband, George. He had been in finance and had a successful early career but had lost his job 10 years previously and was unable to obtain a new one. He was bitter about his lack of success. His resultant irritability caused him to lash out at their 16-year-old son, Adam, centering on his academic struggles. She felt both frustrated but also worried about George, and this limited her ability to confront him about his attitude and behavior.

> Ms. Q: My husband is so morose. I just wish he would do something to try to get back to work, even in a different field. And he doesn't really pay attention to Adam, or if he does, he gets mad at him.
> Therapist: How has Adam responded to this?

TABLE 4–4.   Ms. Q's problems

---

1. Depressive symptoms, feelings of failure

2. Relationship problems with husband and sister

3. Work inhibitions

> MS. Q: It's terrible. He says, "Dad hates me," or, "Dad doesn't care about me." I try to reassure him, but he's been very upset. And he gets angry at his father. He says to him, "Why don't you get a job?" I don't think that's appropriate, but I certainly understand his frustration.
>
> THERAPIST: I assume you've talked to George about these problems?
>
> MS. Q: Oh yes. He doesn't even recognize his moodiness. He even believes he's a good father. I'm worried about hurting him too much, but I tell him he needs to get some form of work if he's not able to get a finance job. Then he gets defensive, and starts attacking me saying things like, "Well what have you accomplished? I don't see you having any successes." And then I feel like a failure again.
>
> THERAPIST: That sounds like a familiar pattern. Like you felt with your sister.
>
> MS. Q: Yes, it does.

Ms. Q reported growing up with a somewhat passive mother and a temperamental, demanding father, who focused on the value of hard work and achievement (Table 4–5). Her father had to work long hours to make money to survive and had to give up his own wishes to pursue an artistic career. When in college she became interested in painting, she suddenly became a focus of her father's rage. He viewed her pursuit of a career in art as "useless" and somehow an insult to him. He remained fixed in this attitude toward her despite early successes with her painting, and they never fully reconciled. He remained cold toward her at family gatherings. She became convinced that she was a failure in her father's eyes and adopted this view of herself.

She acknowledged some anger toward her father but never expressed it directly to him, worried he would respond with a harsh and temperamental attack. To some extent she viewed her sister, a highly successful entrepreneur, as having taken her father's role of being demeaning and critical toward her. Although Ms. Q's mother did not attack her like her father did, she neither intervened when he lashed out nor expressed a different opinion about the patient's behavior or choices. Although she believed her mother did care about her, the patient felt hurt and somewhat unloved by her, as well as angry that she tacitly accepted her father's view. She felt terribly guilty about her fury at the treatment she received and viewed it as further evidence of a sense of "badness" inside her.

> THERAPIST: How might you anticipate you would feel given your father's attacks on you and your mother's unwillingness to intervene? It seems to me it would make sense for you to be angry at them.

TABLE 4–5.   **Ms. Q's representations of self and others/developmental history**

Representations of self and others

Ms. Q viewed herself as "bad," "sensitive," or a failure; others as unresponsive and judgmental. Alternately, she viewed herself as angry and damaging, with others seen as vulnerable and easily damaged.

Developmental history

Ms. Q struggled with her father's view of her as a failure and seeing her artistic efforts as useless. The patient internalized a sense of rage at her father but also incorporated a view of herself as a failure.

> Ms. Q: It's so painful sometimes that it's hard to sort out. I just feel badly about it. And it's also really sad that my mother never made it clear how she felt (*tearful*).
>
> THERAPIST: Well, in addition to tolerating your anger, it also seems like you need to mourn that your relationship with her was not closer.
>
> Ms. Q: Yes, you're right. I guess I always hoped at some point she would come around.
>
> THERAPIST: Did you ever speak to her about it?
>
> Ms. Q: No. I was afraid to. I mean she was clearly avoiding it. And in some ways I was worried to find out what she thought.

Case Example

Mr. N (see Chapter 3), a 42-year-old salesman, reported recurrent bouts of severe depressive symptoms, including intense self-criticism, temper outbursts, alcohol problems, and disruptions in concentration, energy, sleep, and appetite (Table 4–6). Mr. N's episodes would typically be triggered by financial concerns, with intense feelings of being a "fuck up" and failure, even though he had been fairly successful with typical ups and downs of being in sales. Alternately, he felt rebellious with a belief that he did not want to work for a conventional company. A psychiatrist who worked with the therapist prescribed escitalopram for this patient with partial relief of symptoms.

In addition, he had chronic conflicts with his wife and son. He felt that his wife would frequently unfairly attack him for his difficulties with work and his drinking (which he viewed as limited and in control). He experienced marriage as being "like a caged animal." In addition, he would take long trips seeking business opportunities, which also provided relief from tensions at home. He was frustrated that his 15-year-old son spent a significant amount of time in his room playing computer games and smoking marijuana. However, when he asked his son questions about his activities or encouraged him to focus on his homework, his son would become furious. At times he would viciously attack Mr. N, telling him to "stay the fuck out of my life." Mr. N believed that his wife would problem-

---

TABLE 4–6.   Mr. N's problems

---

1. Depressive symptoms, feelings of failure

2. Relationship problems with wife, son

3. Temper outbursts

4. Alcohol binges

---

atically side with his son when he attempted to set limits with him or get him to seek help. He had wanted his son to be able to express frustration, which he had been unable to as a child, but worried he had been too permissive. He would frequently drink heavily after these family conflicts, leaving him irritable and in despair. At these times he would lose control of his temper toward his wife and son, then later suffer intense guilt and self-criticism for these outbursts.

Mr. N reported a background of neglect with his parents, whom he described as deeply involved with their own activities (his father was a successful lawyer and mother worked in the fashion industry), giving little attention to him and his sister (Table 4–7). His parents had increasingly vicious fights beginning when he was age 8, and they divorced when he was 12. His mother essentially left the family to pursue her fashion career and he decided to live with his father. However, as he entered adolescence, his father became increasingly verbally abusive, calling the patient a "loser," often threatening to kick him out of the house. Fights with his father would leave him feeling helpless and like a failure. He noted, however, that things could be just as painful with his mother during his occasional visits with her. Any criticism of her was met with steely withdrawal, sometimes over days, that left the patient feeling frightened, alone, and unloved. He neglected his schoolwork and spent time with a group of boys who were also rebellious, used drugs, and often skipped school. He was "rescued" by a school counselor who recognized his intelligence and supported his efforts to find a good college. When he moved from home to college, he was able to function better, crediting the much reduced "noise" from the vicious conflicts that took place there. He felt a positive reaction from most women but viewed himself as "weak" for seeking this attention.

Traumatic Experiences

As noted in Chapter 3, trauma has a role in the development of a broad range of symptoms and behavioral problems, as well as personality disorders (Casey and Strain 2016; Kessler et al. 2010). In addition, traumatic events, including abandonment, loss, separation, or abuse, can add to a sense of insecure attachment to caregivers, negative representations of self/others, and more disruptive intrapsychic conflicts. Therapists remain alert to the impact of trauma as part of the psychodynamic formulation and the development and persistence of problems.

TABLE 4–7.   Mr. N's self and other representations/developmental history

Self and other representations

He viewed himself as angry and rebellious, focused on aggressive and assertive activities. If not rebelling he viewed himself as weak and a failure. He was unable to bring an empowered sense of self to bear on his experience of himself as a failure. He had a sense of himself as lovable when responded to by women but as weak in seeking attention.

Others were experienced as harsh and critical, withdrawing in response to his rebellion and attention seeking. With some women he felt love, care, and responsiveness.

Developmental history

His parents were neglectful. His father was abusive, with humiliating attacks on him for being a failure. The patient languished at school, almost flunking out. His mother was disengaged, self-focused, and withholding when angry.

Case Example

Mr. R, a 28-year-old securities analyst, presented with depressive symptoms and significant guilty feelings regarding his relationship with his girlfriend. Preceding the onset of his depression, he became sexually involved with another woman after an episode of drinking. He was struggling with intense self-criticism about having betrayed his girlfriend at the time he entered treatment. He decided to reveal the episode to her, and after a period of time and many discussions she decided to continue the relationship with him. This effort led to some reduction in his guilty feelings, but his depressive symptoms persisted. During the initial evaluation he had mentioned how a friend of his in high school had committed suicide but focused on his current relationship difficulties. Several sessions into treatment he revealed that he wanted to share his struggle with depression with others but was embarrassed about doing so. He mentioned that his friend had not revealed his depressive or suicidal feelings.

In this context, the therapist asked him to elaborate about what had happened with his friend. Mr. R revealed that he and Sam were very close friends in high school. Indeed, he was the last one to see him prior to the suicide. Neither the patient nor any of their friends had any idea that Sam was suicidal or even depressed. The patient was completely stunned when he heard the news. After the suicide Mr. R spent significant time with Sam's distraught family members. Mr. R's final exams and college application process were disrupted by his focus on his friend's suicide, and he felt "numb" for several months. He and his girlfriend at the time broke up, and their group of friends drifted apart. As he began to recover, he became close to a new group of friends at college and reengaged in his studies. In addition to his sadness, he realized that he struggled with anger at his friend for having done this to his family and others.

MR. R: I get now I'm mad at him, but I'm having difficulty with feeling that way.

THERAPIST: Can you say more about that?

MR. R: I feel some guilt, but he hurt his friends and family so much. If he had just said something we could have helped him.

THERAPIST: Well that's not clear. You really don't know what help he might have been getting. But it is painful and frustrating that you didn't know. But you had just mentioned not revealing your depression to others and you're angry at your friend for not having said anything.

MR. R: Yes, I didn't realize that connection. And when I have talked to people, I have found it helpful. And this session has been helpful. I guess I've never really told anyone how terrible that experience was.

Intrapsychic Conflicts

Elucidation of intrapsychic conflicts represents a core aspect of the psychodynamic formulation and identifying them for patients is a key part of PrFPP. These conflicts include typically unconscious wishes or fantasies and the internalized prohibitions and emotional reactions that these fantasies trigger, such as guilt or anxiety (Freud 1926/1959). Two wishes can also be experienced as contradictory and in conflict, such as to care for and desire to hurt another person. Although unconscious conflict is universal, individuals can struggle with more severe forms that cause psychopathology and a variety of problems.

Certain core conflicts are relevant to dynamics of many disorders and problems. Wishes to hurt or damage others, dependent wishes, and sexual fantasies are common sources of conflict. Fantasies of outdoing, harming, or dominating others can create conflict in various ways:

1. These wishes can cause anxiety, with fears of disrupting important attachment relationships and triggering retaliation. This dynamic is common in psychiatric disorders, including anxiety disorders and Cluster C personality disorders, in which patients often have a sense of fearful dependency on others that increases the perceived danger of angry fantasies or wishes to harm.
2. Aggressive wishes toward others will often trigger guilt about harming or damaging others who are also needed and loved. This conflict can lead to anger being turned inward with self-criticism or self-punishment. This dynamic is common in depressive disorders.
3. Conflicted anger can be projected onto others, who are then perceived as more attacking or rejecting than they may be in reality, intensifying anxiety, depression, and interpersonal problems.

Core wishes to be cared for or intimate can trigger fears of rejection or intrusion and engulfment by others. Sexual wishes can trigger guilt and anxiety if there is a sense that these fantasies are difficult to control or inappropriate. Additionally, sexual wishes may combine with conflicted wishes for intimacy or aggressive fantasies, leading to conflict about the accompanying sexual fantasies. This is not an exhaustive list; the therapist should attend to the particular nature of the emergence of patients' conflicts as they relate to specific problems.

Defenses

Defense mechanisms (see also Chapter 2) represent the ways in which patients characteristically defend themselves from painful affects, negative perceptions of themselves and others, or threatening unconscious fantasies (A. Freud 1946). Defenses typically operate outside of conscious awareness, and an important therapeutic task is helping patients to be aware of how these defenses operate. Several defenses play a role in attempting to manage angry feelings and fantasies, noted to be a source of conflict as above. These include *reaction formation*, in which the individual adopts a compensatory submissiveness or caretaking of others toward whom they are actually angry. In the defense of *undoing*, individuals symbolically or verbally take back an angry expression or wish. They might be heard saying of a partner, "I hate him, but I really love him." While such defenses can be found normally or in any disorder, they are quite common in panic and other anxiety disorders, in which the individual is attempting to manage anger and make their attachment feel more secure. In *passive aggression*, individuals express anger indirectly via behaviors such as lateness and withholding. The following vignette provides an example of the operation and approach to reaction formation.

Case Example

Ms. S, a 24-year-old public relations consultant, became involved with Bob, who was quite needy of her support, because he was depressed about his unemployment and financial difficulties. In therapy she expressed increasing concerns about the relationship; she had become aware of a pattern of becoming involved with men who were dependent on her and then getting frustrated and disappointed with them. When the therapist explored what attracted the patient to Bob in spite of his problems, Ms. S focused on her boyfriend's positive traits, including his intelligence, congeniality, and warmth.

Over time, however, Bob's dependency intensified. He moved in with the patient because of his financial woes and spent much of his time "hanging out" at her apartment, doing little in the way of housework. Ms. S became increasingly depressed. She felt exhausted by Bob's problems, even though she felt she still needed to help him. She became very self-critical about her tendency to get involved with needy men. However, she expressed little direct anger toward him.

> THERAPIST: It seems like you would be more frustrated with Bob! It sounds as if he's really not doing much to earn his keep.
>
> Ms. S: He just really needs help. The problem's mine for getting involved with guys like this. I've got to try to understand more about that.

THERAPIST: I certainly agree with you, but how do you feel about how he's conducting his life at this point?

Ms. S: Well, I guess he could be doing more to help out me and himself. He's not looking for a job, but he could at least clean up the dishes. I mean, I'm supporting him.

THERAPIST: Have you spoken to him about this?

Ms. S: Well, some. But I don't want to get him even more upset. He really feels bad about himself.

Further exploration of the patient's pull toward needy men proved to be of value, allowing a genetic interpretation that further aided the patient's insight. Ms. S's father was distant and critical, a successful entrepreneur who showed little emotion. She described her mother, on the other hand, as emotionally more connected to her, although also self-involved and somewhat depressed. Ms. S believed that when she was needed by others, her attachment would be closer and more intimate. She feared getting angry because she worried that the man might be "sensitive" like her mother and feel injured, disrupting their tie. However, she became demoralized when she felt she was not getting what she needed from her relationships.

As therapeutic work on this issue continued, Ms. S became increasingly aware of her frustration. She decided that she needed to take some action, so she pressed her boyfriend to get a job and find his own place. To her surprise, he responded positively to these suggestions. As he became more independent, their satisfaction with the relationship increased. This interpretation of reaction formation and her access to underlying anger helped resolve her struggles with assertiveness and relationship problems.

Repression is a defense mechanism through which feelings, fantasies, and memories that create conflict, pain, and anxiety are kept from conscious awareness. In dealing with repression, the therapist works to bring affects, thoughts, and memories to consciousness by helping patients to become aware of and feel safer with these mental states. An associated defense, *denial*, also operates to keep painful feelings and fantasies out of awareness.

Other defenses function to ward off low self-esteem. Individuals can counter feelings of inadequacy by *idealizing* aspects of themselves or others with whom they are emotionally connected. This is a common dynamic in patients with narcissistic personality and depressive disorders, in which compensatory idealization can lead to significant disappointment for patients in themselves and others when they are unable to meet expectations. Another common defense in depression is *projection*, in which angry feelings are experienced as coming from others, adding to a sense that others are rejecting, lowering self-esteem.

Somatization is a defense in which impulses and fantasies that are experienced as dangerous are displaced onto the body or worries about one's health. For example, fears of loss of control of impulses can be displaced to fears of loss of control of the body, such as feelings of vertigo or incontinence. Somatic symptoms can also derive from a lack of capacity to identify bodily aspects of emotions, such as those that contribute to anxiety and anger. Mr. P's gastroin-

---

TABLE 4–8.   Mr. P's intrapsychic conflicts and defenses

1. Conflicts about his anger at his father, which was expressed indirectly via rebelliousness against "the establishment"

2. An awareness of his financial dependency and longing for his father's attention, triggering fears of neglect and rejection

3. Denial and repression of his anger, which was expressed indirectly

4. Somatization (gastrointestinal symptoms, emetophobia), which functioned as a way to avoid painful feelings and fantasies

---

testinal symptoms represented both his fears of being out of control and being humiliated.

Dissociation is a mental state characterized by a disruption in the normally integrated functions of behavior, thoughts, consciousness, feelings, memories, and identity, in which patients feel disconnected from others, reality, or their own emotions. For example, an individual may speak of a traumatic event while consciously experiencing an absence of emotion or sense of numbness. Alternatively, individuals can experience anxious or depressive symptoms clearly related to trauma but not consciously make the connection. Dissociation often functions as a defense in an unconscious effort to mitigate the pain, memories, and associated emotions of traumatic experiences. Pervasive numbing can be an unconscious means of avoiding the distress associated with the trauma or the experience of profound loss or guilt.

Splitting represents an important defense often found in borderline personality disorder (see Chapter 7) or those exposed to severe trauma. In this defense the individual unconsciously protects others from his or her rage by separating "all good" from "all bad" others who are deserving of contempt and aggression. These black-and-white perceptions are typically dissociated, interfering with the capacity of the individual to integrate them. One outcome of this defense is sudden shifts from highly positive to highly negative perceptions of others and associated mood lability. Poor impulse control often results from these intense affects. *Acting out*, also common in personality disorders, involves defending against intolerable feelings and fantasies through impulsive action, such as sexual or aggressive behavior, or substance abuse.

Mr. P struggled with conflicts about his anger at his father, which was expressed indirectly via rebelliousness against "the establishment," lack of attention to schoolwork, having long hair, and playing in a band (Table 4–8). An awareness of his financial dependency and longing for his father's attention triggered fears of neglect and rejection. In terms of defenses, he *denied* and *repressed* his anger, which was expressed indirectly. His *somatization* (gastrointestinal symptoms, emetophobia) functioned as a way to avoid painful feelings and fantasies.

TABLE 4–9.   Mr. Q's intrapsychic conflicts and defenses

---

1. Conflicts about her anger at her parents, husband, and sister, and anxiety and feelings of guilt because she believed her anger was "inappropriate" and feared retaliation for expressing it

2. Feelings of guilt because she feared her anger would be damaging, linking any anger with her father's vicious temper

3. Directing her anger at herself and attacking herself as a failure, and accepting her father's and sister's attitudes toward her, to protect her from her anger toward them

4. Being nicer when she was angry at others (reaction formation)

5. Being late for meetings with her sister, indirectly expressing her frustration with her (passive aggression)

6. Denial of her own anger and projection of it onto others, believing they rejected her for being "a failure"

Ms. Q struggled with conflicts about her anger at her parents, husband, and sister (Table 4–9). She felt anxious and guilty because she believed her anger was "inappropriate" and feared retaliation for expressing it. She felt guilty because she feared her anger would be damaging, linking any anger with her father's vicious temper. Her anger would become self-directed, attacking herself as a loser. Viewing herself as a failure protected her from her anger and caused her to accept her father's and sister's attitude toward her. Ms. Q would often end up being nicer when she was angry at others, unconsciously using the defense of *reaction formation*. She assumed most of the financial burden and chores in the relationship with her husband, despite his unwillingness to look for a job. She said, "I don't say anything about paying for things because he feels bad enough about himself already." The defense of *passive aggression* emerged in Ms. Q's lateness for meetings with her sister, indirectly expressing her frustration with him. In the defense of *projection*, Ms. Q would deny her own anger and also project it onto others, believing they rejected her for being "a failure."

Mr. N was caught in a whirlpool of anger and intense self-criticism (Table 4–10). He experienced his rages as highly damaging and guilt-provoking, as he linked them to his father's behavior, leading them to become self-directed. His anger was also expressed via rebellion, which often resulted in damage to himself. Financial concerns and lack of active business opportunities were "currents" that led him into the whirlpool, as he would feel both frustrated and intensely self-critical. He internalized his father's intensely negative attitudes toward himself. He believed his longings would be met with rejection and neglect, leading to a painful experience of feeling unlovable.

A key defense that Mr. N demonstrated was *identification with aggressor*, in which he connected his self-image with those in power, particularly his father.

TABLE 4–10.   Mr. N's intrapsychic conflicts and defenses
1. Angry feelings that were experienced as highly damaging and guilt-provoking, as he linked them to his father's behavior, leading them to become self-directed
2. Expression of his anger via rebellion, which often resulted in damage to himself
3. Internalization of his father's intensely negative attitudes toward himself, and a belief that his longings would be met with rejection and neglect, leading to a painful experience of feeling unlovable
4. Linking of his self-image with those in power, particularly his father, and feelings of intense guilt and self-criticism in connecting his feelings and actions to his father's damaging, bullying behavior (identification with aggressor)
5. Turning to drinking to salve his painful distress, which would only increase conflicts with his family and lead them to criticize his behavior, leading to anger and guilt and the feeling that he was being punished by their withdrawal (acting out)

However, he would then feel intense guilt and self-critical in linking his feelings and actions to his father's damaging, bullying behavior. Mr. N was also prone to *acting out*, such as turning to drinking to salve his painful distress. The drinking, however, would increase conflicts with his family, and lead them to criticize his behavior. He would then feel angry, guilty, and punished by their withdrawal, tending to minimize the impact of drinking.

Mentalization Deficits

Mentalization is the capacity to conceive of and interpret behaviors and motives in self and others in terms of mental states (Busch 2008; Fonagy and Target 1997). Therapists work to determine mentalization difficulties that contribute to specific problems. Mentalization is most likely to be disrupted in the context of intense attachment relationships, impairing the ability to communicate about needs and wishes. Many problems result from a misinterpretation of the behavior of others, or anticipation of certain actions and attitudes. An improved comprehension of the motives and communication of others can aid in relief of these problems. For instance, patients who experience critical behavior from others can be helped by recognizing that others may be acting on the basis of their own problems, rather than a difficulty of the patient's.

Ms. Q's most significant mentalization difficulties arose in her relationships with men to whom she was closely attached. For example, she tended to accept her sister's intense criticism of her as correct. At other points she was quite angry at her attitudes, yet had difficulty thinking about what factors led her sister to be so judgmental toward her. When the therapist explored this with her, she was able to consider what led to her sister's rigidity.

> THERAPIST: Have you thought about why your sister is so judgmental?
>
> Ms. Q: Usually not. I guess as I think about it, she seems to think she always knows the right way to do things.
>
> THERAPIST: Do you have an example of this?
>
> Ms. Q: Well, when it comes to money, she thinks if you have more you must be a superior person. She's critical of my art career because I don't make as much money as she does in business. And she doesn't recognize how her background helped her to be financially well off. She doesn't empathize with those who struggle financially because of their history.
>
> THERAPIST: It sounds like you're fairly critical of her attitude.
>
> Ms. Q: As I think about it, her attitude is very reminiscent of my father's. And I don't agree with it at all. I don't think people are better because they work in finance. In some ways I think they often ignore things that are very important to people, like art and culture.
>
> THERAPIST: Well, it's interesting then that you often accept her critiques of you.
>
> Ms. Q: I guess I do globally, but thinking about this one I shouldn't accept it.

Engaging Ms. Q's mentalizing capacity enabled her to consider how her sister focused on money as the only sign of success and struggled to empathize with others who lacked privilege. At that point, her sister's attitude could be clearly connected with her father's. Subsequently she became able to apply this way of thinking to her husband's irritability and considered that her husband's own feelings of inadequacy could lead him to attack her presumptive "failure."

The mentalizing capacities of Mr. P and Mr. N were disrupted by negative expectations of others, leading to a rigid conception of others' motives and feelings. Mr. P's anxiety about others attacking him interfered with his capacity to consider their motives, increasing his anticipation of negative judgments. For example, he would fear that his own associates might be looking to criticize his behavior, not recognizing that they often were fearful of him or hoped to impress him. Mr. N's self-loathing and feelings of failure led him to a presumption that others similarly viewed him as a failure and would reject him for that reason. Working on mentalization skills helped these patients to consider that others might have different attitudes or feelings from what they anticipated, including positive ones.

Interventions Based on the Psychodynamic Formulation

As described throughout the description of PrFPP, the psychodynamic formulation provides a guideline for developing interventions. An overview of interventions for Mr. P, Ms. Q, and Mr. N to address their problems based on the formulation is presented below.

Interventions for Mr. P

Representation of Self and Others

The therapist worked to challenge the patient's persistent childhood sense of inadequacy with his adult view of himself as capable. The therapist examined the patient's unrealistic expectation that others would criticize and attack him, based on his father's judgmental behavior and temper.

Developmental Factors

The therapist worked to link the patient's fears and feelings of inadequacy to his father's demeaning intrusions and the overall neglect he experienced.

Intrapsychic Conflicts

The therapist identified the patient's conflict about feeling rebellious and angry, triggering guilt and fears he would be isolated and rejected as a punishment.

Defenses

The therapist elaborated the function of somatization: the experience of danger coming from body represented feared damage from his feelings and fantasies, along with a plea for help from others.

Mentalization Deficits

The therapist worked to ease the patient's sense of threat from others when he perceived them as judgmental and neglectful; he recognized that others have their own independent concerns that he often mislabeled as rejection.

Interventions for Ms. Q

Representation of Self and Others

The therapist examined the patient's inaccurate perception of herself as a failure. Therapist and patient recognized how this view was exacerbated when she was angry at her husband or sister and how anger became directed toward herself.

Developmental Factors

The therapist helped the patient recognize that her father's attacking her as a failure based on her artistic interests was unfair and how this contributed to negative perceptions of self and others.

Intrapsychic Conflicts

The therapist helped the patient develop increased tolerance of her anger, reducing the need to direct it toward herself. For example, she could realize that she was entitled to be angry at her sister's criticisms. The therapist indicated that her fantasies of damaging others with her anger were overstated and interfered with confronting problems. They identified that her increased sensitivity to others' judgment stemmed from her father's critical attacks.

Defenses

The therapist and patient recognized her caretaking of her husband was in part a compensatory reaction formation to her conflicted anger. They identified and addressed how passive aggressive expressions of anger exacerbated her problems.

Mentalization Deficits

The therapist helped the patient recognize that her husband and sister struggled with their own issues that led to them being highly judgmental of her. This helped the patient to question the accuracy of such criticisms.

Interventions for Mr. N

Self and Other Representations

The therapist addressed the patient's view of himself as a failure and irresponsible, despite his successful work and entrepreneurial efforts. He worked with the patient's self-view as an angry, dangerous man, contrasting it with his sense of being a good, caring person, integrating dissociated self-representations. They addressed his expectation that others would disregard his needs, considering how others actually responded.

Developmental Factors

The therapist and patient worked to understand the impact of his father's abusive behavior and his mother's self-focus and distancing on his current expectations.

Intrapsychic Conflicts/Defenses

The therapist helped the patient to identify more effective means of expressing anger and sense of power. They recognized how his anger became directed inward, in the form of guilt and self-criticism, as he identified with the aggressor, his father.

Mentalization Deficits

The therapist helped the patient understand that he often misinterpreted others' withdrawal as rejection rather than as benign, based on his feelings of guilt and inadequacy.

References

Auchincloss EL: Psychoanalytic Models of the Mind. Washington, DC, American Psychiatric Publishing, 2015

Bowlby J: Attachment and Loss, Vol II: Separation, Anxiety and Anger. New York, Basic Books, 1973

Busch FN (ed): Mentalization: Theoretical Considerations, Research Findings, and Clinical Implications. Hillsdale, NJ, Analytic Press, 2008

Busch FN, Milrod BL, Singer M, Aronson A: Panic-Focused Psychodynamic Psychotherapy, eXtended Range. New York, Routledge, 2012

Casey PR, Strain JJ (eds): Trauma and Stressor-Related Disorders. Washington, DC, American Psychiatric Publishing, 2016

Fonagy P, Target M: Attachment and reflective function: their role in self-organization. Dev Psychopathol 9(4):679–700, 1997 9449001

Freud A: The Ego and the Mechanisms of Defense. New York, International Universities Press, 1946

Freud S: Fragment of an analysis of a case of hysteria (1905), in Standard Edition of the Complete Psychological Works of Sigmund Freud, Vol VII. Translated and edited by Strachey J. London, Hogarth, 1953, pp 3–122

Freud S: Inhibitions, symptoms and anxiety (1926), in The Standard Edition of the Complete Psychological Works of Sigmund Freud, Vol XX. Translated by Strachey J. London, Hogarth, 1959, pp 75–175

Gerlsma C, Das J, Emmelkamp PM: Depressed patients' parental representations: stability across changes in depressed mood and specificity across diagnoses. J Affect Disord 27(3):173–181, 1993 8478505

Jacobson E: The Self and the Object World. New York, International Universities Press, 1964

Kessler RC, McLaughlin KA, Green JG, et al: Childhood adversities and adult psychopathology in the WHO World Mental Health Surveys. Br J Psychiatry 197(5):378–385, 2010 21037215

Nitta M, Narita T, Umeda K, et al: Influence of negative cognition on the parental bonding instrument (PBI) in patients with major depression. J Nerv Ment Dis 196(3):244–246, 2008 18340261

Parker G: Parental 'affectionless control' as an antecedent to adult depression. A risk factor delineated. Arch Gen Psychiatry 40(9):956–960, 1983 6615158

Perris C, Arrindell WA, Perris H, et al: Perceived depriving parental rearing and depression. Br J Psychiatry 148:170–175, 1986 3697584

Perry S, Cooper AM, Michels R: The psychodynamic formulation: its purpose, structure, and clinical application. Am J Psychiatry 144(5):543–550, 1987 3578562

Silove D: Perceived parental characteristics and reports of early parental deprivation in agoraphobic patients. Aust N Z J Psychiatry 20(3):365–369, 1986 3467716

5

Addressing Problems: A Framework

In problem-focused psychodynamic psychotherapy, the therapist allows the patient to open the sessions with his or her own thoughts and feelings and then works to identify the problem(s) that is (are) the central focus of the session. This chapter provides a framework for how the therapist approaches and focuses on specific problems in a given session, weaving in the assessment, formulation, and interventions discussed in prior chapters. The therapist relates the patient's current difficulties to aspects of an evolving understanding of the relevant context, affects and meaning, self/other representations, developmental factors, intrapsychic conflicts, defenses, mentalization disruptions, and personality factors. The therapist and patient then identify how an understanding of the problem and various contributors has been furthered, and what additional approaches to the difficulties can be suggested. The therapist also explores how the elaborated factors may be connected to the patient's other problems, including persistent interpersonal issues.

Examples will be provided as to how the therapist maintains structure but also enables new information to emerge in the course of the session. Identifying and addressing a new problem and the recurrence or persistence of a previously identified problem will be discussed. Additionally, various aspects of the patient's history or the psychodynamic formulation may be the focus of the session, which the therapist ultimately relates back to specific problems and potential interventions.

Identifying and Addressing the Problem(s)

Identifying the Core Problem(s) of the Session

The basis for identifying the problem(s) the patient brings into the session was addressed in depth in Chapter 1. Using the central framework, the therapist explores the context/affects/meanings, history of the problem and developmental factors, dynamics, and self and other representations to elaborate interventions for this particular problem (Table 5–1). If the problem is new, the therapist also considers how it might relate to those problems previously brought into treatment. If the problem has been previously recognized, the therapist identifies new or changing aspects of the problem and further elaborates its history, dynamics, and possible interventions. Finally, if the problem is persistent or recurrent, the therapist and patient work to elaborate factors that may be interfering with its improvement or resolution.

Examining the Context, Affects, and Meaning

As noted in Chapter 3, to better identify contributors to problems, the therapist explores the context, affects, and meanings surrounding the onset or occurrence of the particular issue. To obtain this information, the therapist examines what the patient feels when he/she experiences the problem, as well as what environmental stressors are contributing. In addition, the therapist takes a careful history of the problem to better gain a sense of its origin and development. The meaning of the problem typically relates to the function it serves.

The following case demonstrates how the therapist identified and addressed a new problem that Ms. C (see Chapters 1 through 3) raised in therapy.

Ms. C had focused initially in her treatment on painful feelings of loss she was experiencing in anticipation of her daughter going to college (Table 5–2). Difficulties in the relationship with her husband emerged as an additional problem and a contributor to her fears of her daughter leaving home. As her sadness about her daughter eased with therapeutic work, she focused more on her frustrations at work, including her ongoing struggle with speaking to her boss about a raise. She and the therapist discussed a core dynamic of her struggle: her inability to be assertive or express frustration directly to her boss for fear of disrupting their relationship, a conflict which derived from her experiences with her father. In the following vignette, Ms. C shifted from fears of asking for a raise and brought up a new problem: procrastination and motivational struggles at work:

TABLE 5–1.	Framework for identifying and addressing problems

Identifying the core problem(s) of the session

Examining context, affects, and meanings

Exploring the history of the problem and developmental factors

Elaborating and addressing the dynamics

Addressing mentalization capacities

Addressing factors that are interfering with change

Ms. C: I'm still doing okay about my daughter. I mean she's texting me less, and it's kind of sad, but it's not really preoccupying me. I guess work has been on my mind more.

THERAPIST: What's going on at work?

Ms. C: I haven't made much progress there. I'm still struggling.

THERAPIST: I know we've talked about your difficulties asking for a raise. Is that what's troubling you?

Ms. C: No. Not really. I haven't talked to you about this, but I really procrastinate. I don't get around to the work I'm supposed to be doing.

The therapist proceeded to ask for clarification and examined the context and history of this problem:

THERAPIST: Do you have some examples of that?

Ms. C: Yes, I have a good example. I'm supposed to be working on a campaign of a client who contacted me. It actually would help my case for a raise with the boss if I finished it. But I just haven't been working on it. They emailed me yesterday and asked how it was going. I said, "Oh, it's coming along. I should have something soon." But I'm not doing it.

THERAPIST: What goes through your mind as you think of working on it?

Ms. C: Well, I'm not sure exactly what to do. I have ideas, but I can't decide which one I should pick. I feel I'm going to pick the wrong thing and they won't like it. It's not that I don't have the talent. Other people just present their ideas and they aren't very good, but they get them out there and they're accepted.

Ms. C subsequently described how she had lost confidence in her work, leading her to avoid generating ideas for ad campaigns. In this regard her insecurity, which had been described in social situations, was also found to have emerged with her job. Rather than addressing her procrastination, she had been handing over the clients' work to her colleagues. Alongside her decline in motivation, she became less interested in developing the campaigns. Her lack of effort increased her feelings of incompetence, leading to a vicious cycle of feelings of inadequacy, loss of interest, and decreased motivation on her projects.

TABLE 5–2.   Ms. C's problems
1.   Anxious and depressive symptoms
2.   Intense sadness about her daughter going to college
3.   Feelings of inadequacy and low self-esteem, associated with social anxiety
4.   Frustration with her husband, boss, and work
5.   Difficulties with assertiveness
6.   Newly identified: motivational problems

Exploring the History of the Problem and Developmental Factors

The therapist works to elaborate further information about the history of the problem as a means to understand its origins, contributors, and functions and develop interventions based on this information. After identifying Ms. C's motivational problem and its current context, the therapist shifted toward obtaining additional history, exploring how her struggles with procrastination had developed.

THERAPIST: Are these problems you have always had?

Ms. C: No, I would say they started about 2 years ago. I've struggled with my confidence sometimes and stalled on the work. A couple of times the account representatives became frustrated with my delays, but I eventually finished the assignment. But I haven't struggled like this before.

THERAPIST: So anything you recall about what happened two years ago?

Ms. C: I know that's when Ajay joined our group. Maybe that had something to do with it?

THERAPIST: I know you've felt frustrated with Ajay, but I didn't know it affected your work.

Ms. C: Well, I hadn't thought about it that way, but I know I was irritated about the attention the boss was giving him.

THERAPIST: Can you say more about what frustrated you?

Ms. C: I know that my work is better than his is. But it's kind of weird. I feel that because the boss thinks he's good, maybe he is. Maybe he's better than me.

THERAPIST: I know this insecurity has contributed to stalling your work and asking for a raise. But I think your anger might also be affecting you. Maybe you're expressing it in part by procrastinating! [suggesting the defense of passive aggression]

Ms. C: Hmm…I don't really experience it as related to my anger.

THERAPIST: You may not be aware of it. But we know you're quite wary of expressing your anger directly. So maybe this is an indirect protest.

Ms. C: Oh, I see. Well, if that's the case I'm not sure what to do about it.

THERAPIST: Well, first we'll see if other evidence emerges that your anger is contributing.

As described in Chapter 3, the therapist explores the patient's developmental history to further identify factors that contribute to the current problems and addresses how awareness of these factors might ease the patient's problems. In an example of this approach with Ms. C, the therapist examined whether there was any additional information in her past that might shed more light on her motivational difficulties:

THERAPIST: Do you recall any prior times you struggled like this?

Ms. C: In college, after I was so disappointed about what happened in the application process. I think we've spoken about this some.

THERAPIST: Yes, but I think this is a good time to revisit what happened in greater depth, because it may help us better address your difficulties now.

She recalled her frustration when her father would not get involved in a disciplinary problem Ms. C had experienced in high school (see Chapter 3). When she attended a party where students were drinking, the police were called by a neighbor, and the students at the party were disciplined by the school. Although she had had only one drink, she received the same punishment as other students. She believed that the incident was a "black mark" on her record and that it affected her counselor's motivation to get her into college, sharing, "He seemed kind of indifferent toward me after this happened." She told her father about the incident and believed he should have made efforts to get the sanction removed or speak to the counselor about his disengagement. However, her father only responded, "You shouldn't have been hanging out with that crowd." Ultimately, she had to attend a college low on her list and not consistent with her academic performance.

When she got to college Y, she felt that she did not fit in well there and did not find the academic program very challenging. She struggled with her motivation throughout college and had a mediocre academic record. She acknowledged that she had remained angry at her father's attitude toward her efforts and blamed him for her disappointment in school.

THERAPIST: That sounds quite a bit like your situation now. Except your disappointment and frustration are with your boss rather than your father.

Ms. C: I guess there are some similarities. But my boss is not mean like my father.

THERAPIST: That's true. But you're angry at him for not giving you a raise and your motivation is disrupted in a similar way to college.

Ms. C: I see what you're saying.

Elaborating and Addressing the Dynamics: Developing a Psychodynamic Formulation

The therapist works to elaborate self/other representations, developmental history, conflicts, defenses, and mentalization issues that contribute to the patient's problems in the form of a psychodynamic formulation (Perry et al. 1987) (see Chapter 4), providing an additional framework for addressing problems. In the case of Ms. C, the therapist had been working with the patient on her conflicts about her angry feelings and fantasies, particularly with authority figures. With the material that emerged when exploring Ms. C's motivational difficulties, the therapist was able to make some conjectures about how this problem related to her dynamics.

THERAPIST: I believe that your motivational problems are related to your disappointment and anger at your father regarding his behavior toward you. You don't feel safe expressing your anger directly, so you enact a sit-down strike. And I think you tend to see the boss the same way, and it's similarly affected your motivation.

Ms. C: That's an interesting idea. I know he's different from my father, but maybe just because he's the boss? I don't feel that angry at him now.

THERAPIST: Yet you've said you feel frustrated that he favors your colleague and that you fear his reaction to your asking for a raise.

Ms. C: That's true. I guess I have trouble acknowledging that I react to him like my father because he's not mean. But he certainly hasn't been supportive since Ajay came along. Maybe I'm angrier at him than I thought. He has been unfair in the way he's handled this.

THERAPIST: If so, you might be more scared of your own anger than you realized. It could lead to you expecting him to retaliate even though that's not what he's done in the past.

For Ms. C then, this exploration enabled a better understanding of her motivational struggles and additional dynamic factors that contributed to her inhibitions. Fears of expressing anger led to a defensive, passive aggressive lack of accomplishment of work as a form of "protest," which then triggered feelings of inadequacy and low self-esteem. The result was that she would not take charge and procrastinate instead, ultimately adding to her feelings of inadequacy about her job. The therapist worked with her to help her better tolerate and express her anger directly, enabling her to avoid expressing it passive aggressively and toward herself.

Addressing Mentalization Capacities

The therapist works in an ongoing way to develop the patient's mentalization capacities to address problems (Busch 2008; Fonagy and Target 1997). This ability helps patients to reassess representations of others, including their anticipated responses. This approach was used to address an episode of intense social anxiety and humiliation described by Mr. P (see Chapter 4).

MR. P: I had an episode last week. I was on a train, and of course I'm always somewhat anxious. I had purchased a sandwich and was unsure whether I should try to eat it or not on the trip. I took a bite of it, and frankly it smelled like shit. I began to feel dizzy and sweaty and I got up to go to the bathroom. Next thing I knew I was on the floor of the aisle of the train with two doctors checking me and asking, "Is this okay? And is that okay?" I got up and sat in my seat. But I had to be escorted out at the next station, and everyone was looking at me. I assumed they were thinking, "What's wrong with him?" or "He delayed our trip." I felt totally ashamed and humiliated. The doctor was nice about it. She said, "I've seen this happen twice before. The last one was a football player." I said, "I really appreciate your saying that," but it didn't help much.

THERAPIST: I think one thing that stands out is how much you anticipate others being critical or judgmental. You tend to presume that's how people are responding. The doctor's caring response seems like a surprise to you.

MR. P: I'll have to chew on that one for a bit. I do really expect a negative judgment. It brings to mind the last time I had an episode like this.

THERAPIST: What happened then?

MR. P: I was waiting for the train and passed out and vomited on myself. A guy looked at me and just ran away. He was probably thinking, "That guy must be really drunk. I have to get out of here." I took my shirt off and walked home in a T-shirt. Again I was really embarrassed. But no one really noticed. I guess a lot of guys walk around in T-shirts.

THERAPIST: Here again you believed that the other person was being very judgmental. It sounds as if the guy waiting for the train got frightened, but we don't know what he was thinking. You assumed he thought you were drunk. Just like you assumed the people on the train were mad at you or judgmental. Frankly, this sounds like the kind of criticism you expected from your father when he assumed you were being lazy and attacked you. This pattern was a core part of your relationship.

MR. P: Yes, because otherwise he was kind of on his own. He thought it was more important to be a ladies' man than a father or husband. After my parents separated he had series of girlfriends. He would get mad if I tried to reach him and the girlfriends certainly didn't want me around. I do anticipate others being judgmental.

THERAPIST: Or rejecting.

MR. P: That too.

THERAPIST: You expect them to be judgmental of you for experiencing a loss of control. You equate needing help with being a bad person who should be judged or abandoned. Not as someone who has a problem and needs to be helped. And you expect others now to respond like he did.

MR. P: But my wife was caring and concerned, trying to understand how I fainted. And yet I still focus on the negatives. And it's far reaching. Even at work I keep thinking how I'm going to be in trouble with the boss. Even though I really do fine at work and I have no reason to think he'll be mad at me. How do I fix this?

THERAPIST: I think when you feel a loss of control or in need of help you should consider that you anticipate negative judgments from others and instead consider evidence to the contrary. Also keep in mind that the negative expectations stem from your father's criticism and judgment.

MR. P: I'll certainly think about those things. I know I also feel ashamed. But I think that shame is really wrapped up in how I expect others to respond.

Addressing Factors That Are Interfering With Change

The therapist uses the psychodynamic formulation to address factors that are interfering with the patient's capacity to make changes when confronting problems. Problems often persist because they have a variety of contributors and functions. It can be useful in these instances to have the patient imagine what things would be like if they did not have a particular problem. This approach can help to identify what the patient fears as he or she considers change.

Ms. C continued to be frightened about addressing problems with her boss. To determine what else might be scaring her, the therapist wanted to further explore what contributed to her fears:

THERAPIST: Now that we understand that your struggle with motivation is wrapped up with your anger at your boss, we need to consider what else may relieve your anger and lessen your fears about expressing it. We know you are frightened about addressing your frustrations with your boss directly, but we don't fully understand what you are worried will happen. Perhaps we can explore what it would be like talking to your boss and what you would say to him?

Ms. C: It's scary to talk about asking for a raise, but I could try. I'm afraid he will get mad and threaten my job.

THERAPIST: Well, that is a scary idea. Have you asked for raises before?

Ms. C: Yes, twice. One time was successful; the other not. But he wasn't angry.

THERAPIST: Has he gotten very angry at you before?

Ms. C: Only when I threatened to quit when we were fighting about how to handle an account.

THERAPIST: So none of these instances suggest asking for a raise would cause a disruption with him. What makes you think he will get mad now?

Ms. C: Well, I've seen him get very upset when he's pushed about money, particularly when clients don't want to pay fully for their projects. He can get really mean, like threatening them with lawsuits.

THERAPIST: Yes, but you're obviously not in that position.

Ms. C: But I don't want to be wrong about it. I also found out he was giving certain accounts to Ajay without discussing them in the group, which is not how we usually do it. Maybe I could bring that up instead of just directly saying I don't get paid enough. But what if he says, "Ajay needs more accounts" or "I think Ajay's better than you are"?

THERAPIST: I guess that's possible. We can't always predict what will happen in such a discussion. However, I do believe that you transfer your fears about your father to him.

Ms. C: It's funny you bring that up. My father made some nasty comments to my daughter about the college she's going to, and she was really hurt and angry. She wants me to confront him about it.

THERAPIST: And how do you feel about that?

Ms. C: I've been putting that off as well. I've kind of stopped calling him.

THERAPIST: What are you afraid of?

Ms. C: I feel that it would lead to a big disruption. I'm scared that he will just not be willing to see us anymore. And that's also going to be a problem for my daughter, because she loves seeing her grandmother.

THERAPIST: That sounds very similar to your fears about your boss.

Ms. C: I see what you're saying. They do sound similar. Although with my boss my job could be at risk.

THERAPIST: I believe you're overestimating the danger of these disruptions occurring because it's so frightening to you to feel cut down or disregarded by your father. And you have similar fears with your husband. It's almost like bringing up any concerns you have is a threat to your close relationships.

Ms. C: I know my mother is an exception. But otherwise that's pretty much true. But it's terrible because then I just end up stewing about things. So I'll try to discuss the accounts with my boss first. He might get annoyed, but I don't think he would be furious about that.

Addressing a Previously Identified Problem That Has Persisted or Recurred

If a problem being addressed has already been identified, the session can focus on additional understandings of the context, affects, and meanings, including why the problem persists or has recurred. Additionally, there can be additional elaboration of contributing past events, dynamic factors, or limitations in mentalizing ability (Table 5–3). In each case the therapist brings the discussion back to the problem and the relevant psychodynamic formulation. Furthermore, a link can often be made between further understanding of the problem and other difficulties that have emerged during treatment. The following case examines the recurrence of a previously chronic problem.

Case Example

Ms. T was a 32-year-old woman originally presenting with panic disorder, which steadily resolved over several sessions. The panic attacks were found to have developed in the context of frustration with her boss, whom she believed was blocking her promotion, and her husband, whom she felt was unresponsive to her needs. She yielded to her husband's wishes to spend a significant amount of time in his home office to develop a new business. During this time, however, she became more frustrated about his lack of responsiveness and failure to share chores in the house. She felt lonely and isolated but did not believe she could express her frustrations to him without disrupting their relationship.

Over time, she became increasingly angry and depressed, often blaming herself for their problems. As the therapist explored why she directed her anger inward, the patient revealed that she had been drinking more frequently:

TABLE 5–3.   **Investigation of a previously identified problem**

Additional exploration of historical origins and developmental factors

Further elaboration of the psychodynamic formulation

Additional work on mentalization capacities

> THERAPIST: So tell me about your drinking pattern.
>
> Ms. T: I guess I've been drinking more over the last year or so. I usually drink two glasses of wine per night. But over the last few months I have been having a whole bottle, or sometimes a bottle and a half almost every night.
>
> THERAPIST: What do you think led to this change?
>
> Ms. T: Well, that's pretty easy. It definitely started to happen after these terrible fights we have. I can't stand how I feel at those times. The alcohol definitely numbs the rage and loneliness that I feel.

The patient appeared to be using alcohol to ward off painful feelings associated with a core dynamic, in which she felt pressured to respond to the needs of others and believed it was necessary to dismiss her own needs. Therapist and patient were able to identify that her anger about yielding to others triggered significant fears of disrupting her relationships, leading to panic attacks. In addition, she felt lonely and rejected but felt helpless to get others to respond to her. The therapist discussed how drinking was interfering with her access to and tolerance of her feelings and her capacity to address the problems she was having with her husband.

> THERAPIST: I agree that you are using the alcohol to manage your feelings. But it's not really managing them; it's just pushing them away. You'll need to cut back if we're to find ways to better handle your feelings and assert yourself with your husband.
>
> Ms. T: Okay I'll try. I know it won't be easy. I feel such relief when I start to drink, but then I know I feel much worse later on.

Ms. T worked assiduously to significantly reduce her drinking as she tried to better understand and manage her loneliness and rage (though in many instances, struggles with alcohol persist in spite of such efforts and other interventions are required). Her recognition of the sources of her fears led to fewer panic attacks and small advances in her ability to confront her husband. In the context of individual and subsequent couples therapy her ability to express her frustrations increased, but her husband was resistant to making any changes. Whenever she raised her concerns with him, he responded defensively by criticizing her. Ultimately, she decided to move forward with a divorce.

It became clear that in the search for a new partner, she needed to maintain her newfound willingness to communicate her needs. A few months after her divorce, Ms. T met a new man whom she found to be more responsive. Although it was at times a struggle, she was able to develop a relationship with Jeff characterized by a mutual discussion of needs and wishes. She worked with the therapist to identify signs of recurrence in the pattern of yielding to and becoming frustrated with her new partner, as well as in problems with her family. After dating for 2 months, they decided to commit to an exclusive relationship. However, shortly after taking this step, she presented with a resurgence of her old fears and an increase in drinking, though without panic attacks:

THERAPIST: Can you tell me more about what's troubling you?

Ms. T: I'm kind of regretting I made this commitment.

THERAPIST: Why is that?

Ms. T: Well it's uncomfortable for me to talk about, but I notice that I'm much more frustrated with Jeff in the last couple weeks than before.

THERAPIST: What kinds of things are troubling you?

Ms. T: He always leaves his clothes on the floor. If I didn't pick them up, they would just stay there. And he won't help clean up after dinner. That's somehow just my job. It's starting to remind me of my ex.

THERAPIST: What feels uncomfortable about telling me?

Ms. T: I feel like they're just regular complaints that you would find with a married couple. I don't get why they're bothering me so much. It's kind of embarrassing.

THERAPIST: I think we should try to understand more about why that's embarrassing. We know these are very serious matters for you. It's critical for you not to feel stuck in this place where you can't express your feelings. But have you spoken to him about these things?

Ms. T: No. I mean they just started bothering me. I would be uncomfortable bringing them up. But I know that's part of my old pattern. I've also been trying to keep my drinking within bounds.

THERAPIST: As you think about talking to him, what would make you uncomfortable?

Ms. T: I'm worried he'll get annoyed. He might say, "Oh now that we're exclusive you decide to start attacking me?" Because I've never mentioned them before.

THERAPIST: There's a couple of issues that might have led these behaviors to trouble you more after making a commitment. It may bring up memories and frustrations from your first marriage. It's also possible that this step triggered feelings that you are obligated to him in some way. This could bring you back to the mode of feeling pressured to respond to his needs and not raise your own concerns. It feels more constricting and frustrating for you.

Ms. T: I do recognize that feeling of, "Oh no. Better not say anything to him." I don't want to go back to that place.

THERAPIST: I think you've noticed how frightened you've been about addressing your needs with others and how much better it's gone when you do bring things up. Certainly this has been the case with Jeff. Discussing problems with him has been very positive.

Ms. T: That's true. I know this can sneak up on me.

THERAPIST: I think it's good to take another look at factors in your childhood that have contributed to this pattern so we can continue to
address these recurrences. And I agree about steering away from
the drinking. You've recognized that it always just creates more
problems for you.

Thus, in the context of a resurgence of her old relationship fears, the therapist and she revisited aspects of her developmental history.

Additional Exploration of Developmental Factors

In exploring Ms. T's background, she described her parents as highly focused
on their own needs ("selfish" and "narcissistic"). The family operated on a pre-
tense that everyone got along well, and any disagreements were unspoken or
denied. Her father, a successful financier and her mother, a lawyer at a major
firm, considered their careers to be primary and often worked late nights and
weekends. To the extent they were involved with the family, they focused on the
patient's troubled brother, who suffered from impulse control and conduct disorder problems. On the few occasions when the children complained about
their parents' absence, they were lectured about how ungrateful they were about
the "very nice life" their parents worked hard for them to obtain.

Elaborating on the Psychodynamic Formulation

With Ms. T's parents, expressing frustration about their attitudes was not tolerated, and maintaining a sense of closeness required submission. Ms. T internalized a view of her own needs as unsafe to express and "bad," as she felt pressured
to yield to the needs of judgmental and demanding others. Recognizing this
pattern of representations and her fear that expressing her anger or needs would
disrupt close relationships had helped Ms. T to increasingly assert herself with
others, including her new boyfriend. Although she had developed the capacity
to operate in a different mode of self/other representations and dynamics, when
her fears recurred, she would shift back to her old representations. The therapist
and she worked to identify her proneness to return to the old reflexive mode,
something she had been unaware of, and to address what triggered it.

In the current instance, commitment to her new relationship led her to feel
constricted and to shift emotionally to these old representations, interfering with
her ability to address her newfound frustrations with her boyfriend. As opposed
to the past, she was more aware of her irritation, which helped to avert panic at-

tacks and limit the recurrence of drinking. Her anger, however, still frightened her, and she would become submissive and fearful. The therapist reminded her that her relationship was built on a mode of give and take of needs and wishes, with each of them able to express their feelings directly. This approach helped Ms. T to recognize that she was misperceiving the threat with Jeff, and she more readily addressed his behaviors. He did get annoyed at first but quickly settled down and worked to respond to her concerns. The therapist used this opportunity to further the work on Ms. T's mentalization skills, as she better understood her tendency to presume others would be critical if she expressed her wishes.

Addressing the Dynamic Formulation When It Becomes a Focus of the Session

Occasionally the focus of the session will be on the patient's developmental history or dynamics, rather than a particular problem. In these instances, the therapist works to further elaborate these factors, but ultimately identifies how they are relevant to that patient's problems.

Case Example

In a session with Ms. U, a 45-year-old woman with panic disorder, major depressive disorder, and dependent personality disorder, the therapist and patient focused on memories that emerged after the prior session and associated conflicts that she struggled with, before linking the information to her current problems.

> Ms. U: I've been thinking about what you've been saying about how I'm frightened of my anger. I had a memory of my mother after we discussed it last time that I'm sure was significant.
> THERAPIST: What came up?
> Ms. U: I remember an incident when I was 11. She was drinking and started screaming at me about my being fat. I was really furious and worried about her. Then I had thoughts about hurting her.
> THERAPIST: Can you tell me more about these thoughts?
> Ms. U: Do I have to say the details about them?

The therapist was aware that such a question was unusual for this patient, indicating she was uncomfortable about these particular thoughts or fantasies. One option is for the therapist to ask the patient what his or her concerns are in revealing the details, potentially elaborating what the patient feels guilty about or a transference fantasy about how the therapist will react. In this case he encouraged Ms. U to disclose the details, while recognizing the struggle she was having:

THERAPIST: I do think it's important. Plus, the fact that you're hesitating to tell me is relevant, because you must be really upset and maybe guilty about having had these thoughts.

Ms. U: Definitely. I mean it's scary and it's embarrassing. Does anyone else have thoughts like these about their mothers?

THERAPIST: I think everyone has had angry feelings toward their mothers. And if the mother has been abusive then these angry feelings can be even more intense.

Here the therapist provided a brief psychoeducational comment to reassure the patient that aggressive feelings and fantasies toward a parent are common and that abuse tends to heighten these feelings.

Ms. U: Well, okay. Because I remembered having urges to hit her and kick her. I felt really guilty and scared. Now I just feel bad, but I'm relieved to hear you say other people might experience these feelings. It doesn't mean they're crazy.

THERAPIST: I think it's important to become more tolerant of the rage you experience. I think it becomes very frightening to you and interferes with your expression of any frustration with your husband and son. I believe you've associated being assertive with these rageful fantasies, and the intense anxiety and guilt you suffer disrupts these efforts.

Ms. U: You think that's part of why I feel like such a jerk even when I get angry normally?

THERAPIST: I think so. Also, you associate any expression of frustration with your mother's abusive rages when she was drunk.

Ms. U: Well, that is helpful. I guess I can see how it inhibits me now that I remembered how enraged I was. I really must have pushed those feelings away.

In this instance the patient and the therapist worked directly with the framework and developmental history to address the patient's problem in the session. The therapist subsequently explored how identification with the aggressor (her connecting her own anger and vengeful fantasies to her mother's damaging rages) created conflicts for the patient in her experience and management of her own anger.

Identifying Personality Factors and Interpersonal Problems

The therapist works to identify personality factors that are contributory to patients' problems (see Chapter 7 for a fuller discussion). The patients in these examples struggled primarily with Cluster C personality issues, including inhibitions and fearfulness in social relationships. Ms. U, for example, had dependent personality disorder (American Psychiatric Association 2013), in part related to her conflicts with assertiveness. She protected against fears of her anger and autonomy by presenting herself as weak and incapable. However, this added to her negative self-perceptions, as she viewed her dependency as humiliating, potentially leading to rejection. Addressing these conflicts helped her to feel safer being assertive and less dependent, as she came to believe her relationships were less vulnerable to disruption.

References

American Psychiatric Association: Diagnostic and Statistical Manual of Mental Disorders, 5th Edition. Arlington, VA, American Psychiatric Association, 2013

Busch FN (ed): Mentalization: Theoretical Considerations, Research Findings, and Clinical Implications. Hillsdale, NJ, Analytic Press, 2008

Fonagy P, Target M: Attachment and reflective function: their role in self-organization. Dev Psychopathol 9(4):679–700, 1997 9449001

Perry S, Cooper AM, Michels R: The psychodynamic formulation: its purpose, structure, and clinical application. Am J Psychiatry 144(5):543–550, 1987 3578562

6

Addressing the Role of Adverse and Traumatic Experiences in Problems

Traumatic events can be significant contributors to patients' problems (Casey and Strain 2016; Kessler et al. 2010). For individuals who suffer from PTSD or other posttraumatic syndromes (American Psychiatric Association 2013) or sequelae, the therapist should address the links between traumatic events and the various presenting difficulties. Patients often perceive or respond to situations in the present as if the traumatic experience is occurring, usually out of awareness. The therapist's tasks include helping patients to recognize how their problems are related to trauma and to build a conception of their thoughts, feelings, and circumstances that is less affected by these events. Several factors relevant to understanding the impact of trauma from the psychoanalytic standpoint are elaborated below (Table 6–1).

As with other problems, posttraumatic perceptions, symptoms, and behaviors are explored with regard to dynamic factors. Common self/other representations include patients' view of themselves as highly vulnerable to damage from others who are seen as abusers, alongside self-perceptions of being enraged at and potentially damaging to others. Developmental history is relevant in understanding how individuals are affected by trauma: Patients with insecure at-

TABLE 6–1.	Addressing the impact of trauma
Proneness to repeating the trauma	
Symptoms of reexperiencing the trauma	
Dissociation	
Phobias	
Identification with the aggressor	
Irritability	
Anxiety and depression	
Somatic manifestations of trauma	
Feeling as if the traumatic experience were occurring	

tachment or who suffered early abuse or adverse developmental events are more susceptible to the impact of subsequent trauma.

In terms of intrapsychic conflict, dangers surrounding anger and dependency are heightened by severe disruptions of trust as well as intense hostility experienced from and toward perpetrators. As will be described, dissociation, identification with the aggressor, avoidance, and somatization are key defenses in patients with posttraumatic syndromes. Mentalization abilities are often disrupted by trauma, because patients have difficulty feeling safe considering the minds of others they perceive as potential abusers.

Proneness to Repeating the Trauma

Individuals are unconsciously prone to repeating traumatic episodes, either intrapsychically or in their behavior or relationship with others, a phenomenon known as "repetition compulsion" (Corradi 2009; Freud 1920/1955). For example, someone who has been abused in childhood may inadvertently become involved in relationships with troubled partners, heightening the potential for recurrence of abuse. Alternatively, individuals may misperceive a relatively benign or moderately problematic situation as if it were a traumatic event or as if they were being abused. A common example of this is a veteran returning to civilian life who experiences loud noises as if they were gunshots or explosions. Another instance would be an employee perceiving a boss's criticisms of not completing work quickly enough as being abusive, when the boss is behaving within the usual range of someone in that position of authority.

Several factors can contribute to repetition of traumatic states. Those who have a history of trauma are likely to anticipate its recurrence, or experience it as recurring, because it was so hurtful or damaging to them; they are highly alert to these potential threats. Additionally, individuals often have an unconscious wish to master or control the traumatic episode(s) in which they felt helpless. They may inadvertently recreate the traumatic experience, fantasizing that there will be a different outcome. For example, they may hope to punish the abuser in a way that was not possible during the original traumatic event. Additionally, particularly when the abuse occurred at the hands of caregivers during childhood or adolescence, patients may experience being abused as a way of being emotionally close, sometimes emerging in the form of a sadomasochistic relationship. The therapist helps patients to recognize how they are continually affected by traumatic events in emotional experiences and relationships and identify how they are inadvertently repeating these episodes.

Case Example

Ms. V, a 36-year-old divorced African American woman, had experienced physical and sexual abuse by her father from ages 7 to 14. She took on the role of the "good child," including yielding to his sexual wishes (typically fellatio), in an attempt to avoid being severely punished (hit with a belt all over her body). Attempts to gain the attention of her mother were usually unsuccessful, as she struggled with alcohol abuse and chronically fought with the patient's father. She grew up believing that others could not be trusted or would ultimately betray her.

Ms. V demonstrated a pattern in her adult life of taking on more of her share of the work in many situations, whether with friends or at the job, hoping to be appreciated for her efforts. However, she would begin to feel taken advantage of, then become increasingly sullen and, usually silently, furious at those whom she hoped to please. They typically did not understand what the patient was angry about and started to withdraw from her. She would then feel increasingly hurt and enraged at them and explode with vituperations in a way they did not expect, leading to disruptions in her relationships. Ms. V felt deeply disappointed and betrayed, but not surprised, saying that others acted as she expected, in a completely untrustworthy and self-interested way.

Another severe problem occurred at her job as an administrative assistant where she worked extra hours for her boss, whom she greatly admired. However, after making a series of inappropriate comments, he attempted to approach her sexually. She became furious at him and aggressively resisted his advances. The boss claimed that he believed her staying overtime was an indication of her interest in him. She did report the incident to Human Resources but felt they gave her the "brush off." Acting out of her hurt and anger, she quit the job then soon became deeply depressed.

The therapist early on identified this pattern of submission to others with the corresponding hope they would appreciate her efforts, followed by an inevitable experience of disappointment, betrayal, and rage when their response was inadequate. In this regard Ms. V repeated the pattern of being the "good girl" to try to "fix" the developmental trauma she experienced but ended up repeating these traumatic events. The patient steadily gained an awareness of this pattern and attempted to avoid getting caught in this cycle.

Symptoms of Reexperiencing the Trauma

Reexperiencing can include flashbacks, involuntary memories, and nightmares that feel as if the traumatic event is recurring. These symptoms can be viewed as another way in which trauma is repeated, creating a sense of powerlessness and lack of control. As with other problems related to the traumatic experience, the therapist explores specific aspects of these symptoms, contexts that trigger them, and their impact on the patient's emotions and perceptions. The symptoms may represent the mind's attempts to develop a coherent narrative or an effort to control or avoid the traumatic experience. Identifying the specific details, meanings, and contexts of the intrusive memories and experiences aids in this integration.

Intrusive memories, flashbacks, and nightmares may also stem from painful conflicted feelings of rage, guilt, and responsibility. For example, an individual may have intrusive, guilt-ridden memories of being unable to save a friend or family member from harm. These preoccupations can represent efforts to undo the trauma ("if only I had done this, he would have been okay") and fantasies of omnipotence ("I should have done this to prevent harm," even though it was actually not possible in the traumatic situation). These fantasies can also be attempts to manage feelings of anger and the pain of loss. Additionally, the patient's rage at the perpetrator, intolerable because of its intensity, can be directed toward the self via guilt ridden fantasies. Helping to untangle these various elements, including identifying the actual limits the individual had to manage the traumatic events, can aid in tolerating the feelings contributing to these symptoms.

Case Example

Mr. W, a 28-year-old veteran, was preoccupied with a fantasy that he should have saved two fellow soldiers from being killed during his tour in Afghanistan. He was highly self-critical for having been a "failure" in this effort. Conflicts in his marriage, an explosive temper, and bouts of drinking added to the difficulties he was having. Exploration of the details of what had occurred in the war indicated that there was little he could do to change the situation:

> THERAPIST: Can you tell me about what happened?
> MR. W: It's very painful for me to recount the story.

In these instances the therapist needs to make a judgment about whether to defer exploration of the trauma or seek more information. Alternatively, the therapist can explore what makes it difficult to talk about the traumatic event. The therapist in this case gently encouraged the patient to describe his experiences:

> THERAPIST: I recognize that it's difficult. Let's see how it goes.
> MR. W: We found out that two of our guys, who were actually close
> friends of mine, had been trapped in another area close to our

unit. We moved quickly to get to them, but then we began taking enemy fire. I wanted to keep going but the commanding officer refused to let us move forward. (*Patient becomes tearful.*) Then we found out they'd been killed.

THERAPIST: That sounds awful. However, I'm not sure how you could possibly have done any more than what you did. What could you do if your CO refused to let you advance?

MR. W: I don't know, but I should have done something. I was with them an hour before they got separated. I actually don't know how it happened. But I should have kept a watch over them.

THERAPIST: Did you have any command over them? Were they your responsibility?

MR. W: Well not officially, but we're supposed to look out for each other. I should have noticed they were missing.

THERAPIST: But it sounds like there was a lot going on that you had to focus on.

MR. W: Oh yeah. We were already taking fire. I was distracted.

THERAPIST: Well, I think we need to try to understand how you continue to blame yourself when there was really nothing you could do. Maybe you want to believe you could have rescued them because it's very painful to accept how helpless you were.

MR. W: That could be, but it doesn't feel that way. Plus, I feel so terribly guilty. I don't know why they didn't survive, and I did. And here I am making a mess of things since I've been back. With my drinking and my temper. My wife is actually frightened of me!

THERAPIST: I think it's essential to explore your intense guilty feelings, because I think in a way, you're continuing to punish yourself through your behavior and self-criticism. And I suspect that you drink in part to try to address the pain you feel.

MR. W: Yes, I do start drinking when this self-loathing ratchets up in my head. It's the only thing that helps for a bit, but then it comes roaring back.

Mr. W's intense guilt was found to have roots not only in the war but also in a history of neglect by his father. He reported that his father often left home for long periods. While he was told that his father was working, he later learned that he was spending time with a series of girlfriends; his mother ignored these dalliances. Mr. W struggled with conflicted rage toward his father for his neglect, which would become self-directed in the form of guilt and self-loathing: He believed he must have been "bad" to be treated this way. He also became angry at himself for what he viewed as being neglectful and irresponsible like his father with his friends who were killed. Identifying the unfairness of these self-attacks was critical in addressing his drinking, which he would do in an effort to temper these painful feelings.

Dissociation

As noted in Chapter 5, dissociation, which often stems from trauma, is characterized by a disruption in links between thoughts, feelings, memories, perceptions, and behavior. These disconnections interfere with patients' capacities to identify the ways in which they have been affected by trauma; the therapist's task includes helping patients to understand this impact and recognize how their problems are related to traumatic experiences. The therapist also identifies how patients defensively avoid recognition or understanding of the impact of trauma via dissociation. Addressing the sources of symptoms can help patients to work through these experiences and link relevant emotions, cognitions, and memories.

As his issues were explored further, Mr. P (see Chapters 4 and 5) recognized his anxiety and insecurity about being attacked or criticized by others were much more extensive than he realized initially.

> MR. P: I've been paying more attention to what I've been feeling. And I think most of the time I'm worrying about what others think of me and whether there is going to be some kind of negative judgment. I worry whether I'm paying enough attention to my wife or she'll be mad at me and whether I'm doing enough work at the office and my boss will reprimand me. We're in a glass office, and if somebody walks by, I think about what I'm doing and what they noticed and whether I'm going to get into trouble.
>
> THERAPIST: So rather than a few situations like we addressed before, it sounds like your worries are much more extensive. Ultimately you don't feel safe around others, and you're always anxious you're going to get into some kind of trouble. It all sounds like you're worried you're about to be reprimanded by your father! And we know that you don't really have to be concerned about your relationship with your wife or your work. You're doing well at work and there's no indication of a problem.
>
> MR. P: It's like a guy leaving Vietnam still fearful of loud noises. I'm still thinking my Dad is about to come in and yell at me for what I'm doing. I didn't notice how closely connected my fears now were to him.
>
> THERAPIST: I don't think you realized how much you still feel those dangers now. I think that's in part because it's as if these dangers were normal to you. The expectation of them happens reflexively even though they're not relevant to how you're doing now.

Mr. P had dissociated his father's punishments from his current expectation of reprimands. Clarifying this connection helped him have both a more coherent narrative regarding the development of his problems and a way to address his irrational fears with others.

Phobias

Although multiple factors can contribute, phobic symptoms and behavior at the level of a disorder are a common outcome of trauma (Busch et al. 2012). The psychological avoidance of painful memories or feelings is frequently accompanied by behavioral avoidance of certain people, activities, or sensory experiences that are linked with traumatic events. Severe forms of phobic avoidance can also derive from adverse developmental experiences with frightening, neglectful, or abusive caregivers. The therapist explores how the fantasy, intrapsychic conflicts, and defenses triggered by trauma contribute to avoidance. Phobic fears are often displaced to places or particular circumstances that symbolically represent the patient's intrapsychic fears.

An initial step of this approach is to identify the probable connections between the phobic behavior and the traumatic or adverse developmental events. In many instances an individual does not recognize the relationship because the link has never been suggested and/or dissociative tendencies or defenses have blocked a conscious connection. Identifying the link is an important step in developing a framework for addressing the problem, such as with the comment: "I wonder if your terror of being trapped in the subway may be related to the way you felt trapped with your mother during her alcohol fueled rages."

After such links and dynamics are identified, the therapist can work with the patient in clarifying that the phobic dangers are not realistic or highly unlikely in the present situation but are derived from past traumatic experiences and internal fears. Therapists can then have the patient imagine the dangers that they fear relative to what they have understood about the origin of their avoidance.

Identification With the Aggressor

Identification with the aggressor (Freud 1936) (see Chapter 2) is often a central element in understanding the impact of trauma on the patient's current problems. In unconsciously employing this defense, the individual identifies with the perpetrator of the trauma or others who have had power and control over them. Such an identification may be experienced in fantasy (e.g., wishes for revenge against or damage to the perpetrator) or enacted with others (e.g., bullying others as one has been bullied). At the same time, wishes to harm others as one has been harmed can create significant guilt, distress, and behavioral inhibition. For example, a mother who was physically abused as a form of punishment as a child can struggle with fears/wishes to harm her own child. In these instances, the parent may inadvertently equate any limit setting with the child as being abusive or neglectful, creating the potential for persistent interactional problems. In addition, patients may enact bullying and aggressive behavior that can damage their own relationships. Because of dissociative processes, patients with this defense may be bullying in certain circumstances and overly inhibited in others.

Case Example

Mr. I (see Chapter 2) perceived and acted as if he were being bullied in an ongoing way by others, as he felt with his father, leading to difficulties with assertiveness and problematic relationships, as well as irritability and depression. Understanding these factors aided the patient in feeling less bullied and more assertive in addressing his frustrations with others. For example, Mr. I became enraged at his children when they did not do what he expected. In an example of dissociative tendencies caused by trauma, he was furious at his own father's controlling and bullying behavior and had vowed not to reenact it with his children, even as he felt the urge to compel them to yield to his authority. Pointing out to Mr. I how his father's attitudes infiltrated his thoughts and feelings aided him in reevaluating his approach to his children and modulating his anger.

> MR. I: I told you that my children are not respectful of me. They don't want to participate in any of the plans that I set up for them.
> THERAPIST: Well, I don't think that's unusual for teenagers. What were your plans?
> MR. I: I wanted to take them to a movie. But they just complained about going. They don't show me any respect.
> THERAPIST: I'm not really sure this is about respect for you. I don't think they want to be caught in the trap.

As noted in Chapter 2, "caught in the trap" was Mr. I's shorthand way of describing the complex feelings he had with his authoritarian father, believing that he had no say in what he wanted to do in his life. His father would override or even demean his ideas for activities his family should do when he was a teenager. For instance, Mr. I was interested in going to museums, to which his father would respond that he was a "sissy" and focus on his brother's sports activities.

> MR. I: So you don't think I should tell them they have to go to the movie?
> THERAPIST: Well, I recognize that in some instances you would have to be firm with them, but I'm not sure about this one. You yourself said that you don't want to put them in a trap like your father did with you. I think sometimes you don't recognize how your father's attitudes or behaviors might emerge in you. You might be identifying with him without realizing it.
> MR. I: I don't really like that idea, but I do recognize that I might bully others in some circumstances. And I don't want to do that with the kids, but I also think I'm afraid to take a firmer stance, because I want everyone to like me.

This statement was shorthand for another impact from his father's bullying and critical behavior. Feeling pressured by his father, he had become aware of needing to please others, for fear of getting rejected or punished. This propensity interfered with his capacity to set appropriate limits with his children and others. He demonstrated the posttraumatic dissociative tendency of fearing asserting himself in certain circumstances while being demanding, irritable, and bullying in others. The therapist helped him to recognize and integrate these conflicting representations. After identifying how Mr. I was being affected by the trauma, the therapist worked with him on integrating the split off aspects and enabling a gradient of response to his children's behavior.

THERAPIST: I think you're talking about two very different reactions to your father's behavior that make it hard for you in dealing with your children. On the one hand you may identify with him in believing you can make them do a specific activity, and on the other hand you may be fearful of setting necessary limits because you feel you need to please them. I think understanding the different ways you are affected would make it easier for you to figure out where to draw the line.

MR. I: I didn't realize I was in such conflict about it.

Irritability

Trauma can heighten difficulties with impulse control in many ways, including difficulties managing sexual impulses, substance use, and anger. Posttraumatic symptoms often include irritability, sometimes alternating with dissociative states. As with other symptoms, patients frequently do not connect angry feelings and behaviors to traumatic and other adverse experiences. Traumatized patients, however, often have underlying rage at perpetrators of the trauma, or others they believe did not protect them. These feelings are frequently displaced toward intimate partners or authority figures not involved in these events. Indeed, it is not uncommon for patients to view the therapist as the abuser, providing an opportunity to explore the impact of trauma and their rage within the therapeutic relationship. Complicating these circumstances, patients may alternate between inhibitions of assertiveness in some situations and overaggressiveness in others, each potentially linked to the traumatic experiences, as noted with Mr. I above. Identifying this variability, connecting the symptoms to the trauma, and identifying alternatives ways of expressing themselves can aid patients in managing their expression of these feelings toward others.

Case Example

Mr. X, a 72-year-old Vietnam veteran, presented with irritability toward his wife. Although he loved her, he would lash out suddenly and unexpectedly, criticizing something relatively benign that she said or did, like saying the dishes were not clean enough. He did not understand what triggered these outbursts and was worried that his wife would get frustrated with these attacks and leave him. However, there was no evidence that his wife intended to do that.

Mr. X stated up front that he had never wanted to be a burden to others. His family, including his parents and six siblings, was impoverished and immigrated from Italy when he was 12 years old. As a child he tried to be the "good boy" by not creating too much trouble for his parents, whom he experienced as overburdened by their chores and financial limitations. Despite being an immigrant, at age 20 he was drafted and sent to Vietnam as a medic. He was so fearful of upsetting his mother that he did not tell her for several weeks that he was in Vietnam. In the war he had multiple traumatic experiences, observing many instances of deaths and mutilations, including of people to whom he was close. However, he persisted after the war in living his life stoically, referring to his attitude as "grin and bear it." He had a successful career as a truck driver and had two children with whom he had good relationships. He had not spoken about his war memories for years until he entered therapy.

The therapist explored how his stoic attitude had helped him to get by in life but also created problems for him. His efforts to not trouble his parents often left him feeling alone and neglected. Not telling anyone about his painful war memories added to his sense of isolation. As the therapist identified the pressure he felt to not burden others, she began to explore the origins of his anger. He talked about the deep pain and distress of his war experiences, including seeing mangled bodies or body parts, as well as the deaths of fellow soldiers. He then revealed that he was deeply angry that, in his view, the war was grossly mismanaged and that many of these deaths were a "waste." He was also upset on his return from Vietnam that soldiers were viewed as "baby killers." His anger at his wife was dissociated from these other experiences.

> THERAPIST: I think we need to consider that your anger toward your wife is related to the anger you felt during the war and after.
>
> MR. X: Well, I hadn't thought about that. It doesn't seem connected. And I try to push that anger out of my mind anyway. You have to grin and bear it, you know.
>
> THERAPIST: But we've also found that grinning and bearing it has created real problems for you; you've often felt isolated and alone with your problems. Did you ever consider talking to her about your experiences?
>
> MR. X: Oh, definitely. But I think she'd be very upset hearing about it. They were very scary and gruesome.
>
> THERAPIST: Does anything in the war remind you of these tensions with her?
>
> MR. X: Well, I hadn't really thought about it before, but one of the things that really terrified me in the war was when we went into the villages. There really weren't any men there. Just women and children. But you could never be sure whether they were friendly or not. At any point they could contact the men, and there could be an ambush. I actually heard about this happening to a platoon we met up with. So I was terrified and furious about being in these situations. And occasionally I'm reminded about that now when I see women who look really troubled or preoccupied. I get scared and angry. But my wife's not really like that. I mean sometimes she seems preoccupied. I don't always know why, and she doesn't like to talk about it. I think it's usually about the kids.
>
> THERAPIST: And is that when you tend to yell at her?
>
> MR. X: Come to think of it, it's definitely one of the times I do it. You think this could be why I get so mad? Because it is way over the top.
>
> THERAPIST: Yes, because sometimes it's hard to connect current problems to traumatic events because they were so painful. Those experiences were terrifying.
>
> MR. X: Yeah, they definitely were.

Anxiety and Depression

Multiple symptoms and problems can develop secondary to traumatic incidents, including anxious and depressive episodes. Anxiety symptoms can often emerge in relation to conflicts or environmental events that are associated with the trauma, and depression can occur in the context of subsequent feelings of helplessness and disruptions in various areas of life functioning.

Case Example

The therapist continued to explore sources of persistent depressive symptoms with Mr. R (see Chapter 4). The patient reported feeling down in the morning, although he would feel better later in the day. He also felt better on the weekends when his girlfriend stayed over. At that point he and the therapist were able to identify that he was more troubled by his symptoms when he was alone.

THERAPIST: So what comes to mind about being alone? Do you feel lonely at those times? You did say you felt better when you were able to talk to others when you were feeling down.

MR. R: Communicating about my depression is less of a problem now. I talked to my siblings about it and they're aware. They're not bringing it up, but I know I can talk to them about it when I need to. So I don't really feel lonely in that regard.

THERAPIST: Well, that's very positive. Anything else about being alone?

MR. R: I have been worried about something happening to my girlfriend or sister when I'm not with them.

THERAPIST: What are you worried might happen?

MR. R: You know there are really crazy people out there. Like you hear about these terrorist attacks. I'd feel terrible if something happened to them and I wasn't around to help them.

THERAPIST: That's a scary thought. Although the risk of being hurt in a terrorist attack is extremely low. The coverage of these events can give people the sense that they're more at risk than they are. But let's try to understand your guilty feelings. You couldn't predict that such an event would occur.

MR. R: Well, I know it's not rational, but I would feel I had failed to protect them.

THERAPIST: Have you had other fears like this?

MR. R: Now that I think about it, I do worry a lot about whether others in my family are okay. My grandparents are kind of old, and I'm particularly close to my grandmother. She's really funny and she would take care of me often as a kid to help my Mom out. She was really nice to have around. But now she has bad arthritis and moves really slowly. Sometimes she doesn't remember things. I wonder how I'll deal with losing her.

THERAPIST: What are you worried about?

Mr. R: That I won't be able to handle it well. That I'll get more depressed again.

Therapist: I can see why that makes you concerned about still feeling down at times or about your symptoms coming back. But it's also important to be aware that that's what we're treating you for. To help reduce this vulnerability. Are there others you're worried about?

Mr. R: Well, actually, my parents. My father lost his appetite a couple months ago. They checked it out and something was wrong with his liver. He doesn't drink so it wasn't that. He seems to be getting better slowly but we were really worried about him.

Therapist: That's pretty scary. I guess we hadn't had a chance to speak about that.

Mr. R: Yeah, I'm not sure why. Maybe we were talking about other things.

Therapist: But that could certainly be a contributor to your depression. It seems like you were dealing with more things upsetting you than we thought.

Mr. R: Yeah. I hadn't considered that.

The therapist then proceeded to explore the history of these fears:

Therapist: How far back does this tendency to worry about others go?

Mr. R: Oh, it's been around a while. A long time. Back to high school.

Therapist: Well, I know in high school you had to deal with your friend's suicide. Sometimes a traumatic event like that will heighten people's worry about the safety of others.

Mr. R: It's strange you mention that. Because I just heard from his brother. We talk every now and then, but it had been a while. It was good to hear from him. He's trying to make the best adjustment he can.

Therapist: Well, that's interesting. So overall you found it a positive conversation?

Mr. R: Yes, but it did bring back some reminders of what happened. How he seemed like such a happy guy. It's still so puzzling.

Therapist: Yes, and that was certainly very sudden. And you felt guilty even though there wasn't any way you could have known about it.

Mr. R: That's true. I see what you're saying. That could have set me off more in terms of worrying about people close to me. It happened out of nowhere! I guess the impact of that experience was greater than I thought.

This vignette is also a reminder of the broad impact of trauma and how it can contribute to a range of problems.

Somatic Manifestations of Trauma

Somatic symptoms and catastrophic fears about them are common sequelae of trauma and often an aspect of dissociation, and can cause distressing anxious preoccupations that can also adversely impact relationships. These symptoms can represent aspects of trauma that have not been translated into the symbolic, verbal sphere (Busch 2017). They may also be somatic memories of the traumatic experience dissociated from other memories of the trauma. In addition, somatic preoccupations can function as a defense against painful or frightening intrapsychic conflicts; patients avoid conscious access to these experiences through a focus on the body. Finally, somatic experiences can also symbolize an underlying intrapsychic conflict (e.g., a patient's experience of an ill or damaged body can serve as a punishment for aggressive wishes). Understanding the link to trauma and relevant dynamics can aid in diminishing these symptoms and associated behavioral difficulties.

Case Example

Ms. Y, a 42-year-old woman, presented with a series of health fears, often involving a pain in some area that she interpreted as cancer. The therapist explored the details and contexts of these fears:

> Ms. Y: I'm really worried that I have cancer.
> Therapist: What makes you think that?
> Ms. Y: Well, I have these headaches, and they've just gotten increasingly more painful.
> Therapist: When do you get them?
> Ms. Y: I typically get them in the evening. It's like a band around my head.
> Therapist: There are a lot of causes for headaches, including stress and tension. In fact, that's not an uncommon presentation of a stress headache. What makes you believe it's cancer?
> Ms. Y: I don't know. I just think it's a brain tumor. I think that's why it hurts so much.
> Therapist: Have you been to see your doctor?
> Ms. Y: No because I've been to him so many times before about all kinds of worries. I'm pretty sure he's sick of me.
> Therapist: Is there anything in particular about the evenings that might trigger the headaches to occur at that time?
> Ms. Y: Well, that's when the kids come home. It is a very stressful time of day.

In exploring these stresses Ms. Y reported significant worries about her children:

THERAPIST: What makes it stressful?

MS. Y: I'm really worried about the kids. Nate, my 8-year-old, refuses to study and do his homework and I get furious with him. I feel bad about how angry I get. But I'm really worried he's going to get behind academically and won't get into a good college. And then he'll have a terrible life.

THERAPIST: Don't you think that's a bit catastrophic? I mean he's just 8 years old.

MS. Y: I don't think so (*tearful*). My brother struggled academically and now he's having a very hard time. And when I get mad at Nate, my head starts to hurt me, and that's when I get worried about cancer!

THERAPIST: It sounds like you have a lot of catastrophic fears. I think we need to do more to try to understand why you're feeling so threatened. Maybe you could tell me a little bit about your family and what that was like for you as a child.

Ms. Y described growing up with a father who was temperamental, critical, and bullying. She described many instances in which he screamed at her for minor errors, leaving her tearful and humiliated. Once when she accidentally broke a plate cleaning up the kitchen, he screamed, "You're horrible. How can you behave the way you do and ruin everything for us? And how will we pay for a new plate?" The patient and her mother and brother formed a close alliance to attempt to provide some protection from her father, but her mother was unable to stop her father's bullying and harsh attacks. She did get some solace from being the leader of her group of girlfriends at school. Although she was able to be fairly successful academically and obtain a good job as an administrator, her brother struggled with drug use and worked intermittently, unable to maintain a job for very long.

Using this information the therapist was able to explore some of the issues with her son.

THERAPIST: So I can see more about what might worry you about your son. Have you thought about your brother when you get anxious about his performance in school?

MS. Y: Yes, definitely. It's terrible what happened with Martin. And he still struggles now. He's married with a kid, but he's barely able to support his family. It's so sad because we were so close as kids. I always tried to help him (*tearful again*).

THERAPIST: I think it's important to recognize that Nate's having a very different upbringing from your brother. It seems like you're assuming that any difficulty now will lead him to behave like your brother based on the trauma the two of you grew up with. Can you say more about your guilt about getting angry at him?

Ms. Y: Yes (*tearful again*). I know he's just a kid but it gets me so mad. Why can't he just get his work done instead of fighting with us?

THERAPIST: Do you worry that when you get angry, you're being like your father?

Ms. Y: Kind of. It is so terrible to yell at a kid like that!

THERAPIST: One important difference is that you recognize your anger is a problem and you're working to control it. But I think your worries about your head may come from fears and guilt about losing your temper. You feel your temper is out of control and damaging, like how you saw your father. A cancer is also out of control and damaging.

Ms. Y: I don't know. I'm still really scared. But I had an MRI just a few months ago, and they didn't see anything. I know that realistically a tumor couldn't have developed since then.

The therapist indicated that Ms. Y was struggling with identification with the aggressor, and her irritation with her son triggered conflict that was intolerable for the patient. The therapist realized that Ms. Y was not quite ready to take in all of what he was saying about her bodily fears, but it was a beginning step to having her consider that her somatic concerns were of emotional origin in part linked to her early trauma. The therapist also considered that Ms. Y might be unconsciously punishing herself for her anger but felt that raising this notion at this point would overload the patient.

Feeling as If the Traumatic Experience Were Occurring

Patients with posttraumatic syndromes will often experience situations as if the trauma were recurring, adding to the intensity of their angry, anxious, or depressive reactions to the current circumstances. A veteran believing a loud noise to be an explosion would be a manifestation of this phenomenon. Oftentimes, however, patients perceive social situations that may be relatively benign or somewhat fraught as a recurrence of a traumatic situation, greatly intensifying their emotional reactions and potentially disrupting their relationships. Patients often feel trapped or stuck in these situations, believing escape to be necessary but impossible.

Ms. Y was furious at her sister-in-law, who she believed kept her brother away from the family and also limited access to her nephew. She felt that her behavior was very hurtful and damaging to the family. She complained to her brother, but he responded that she was making a big deal out of nothing, refusing to acknowledge the patient's concerns. She became more furious but also felt guilty about getting angry at him, worried that she would exacerbate his drug problem. She complained to her mother, telling her that if they were going to behave this way, and keep their son away from them, they should refuse to visit the nephew.

> THERAPIST: How did your mother respond to that?
>
> Ms. Y: She doesn't get it. She said, "I can't not go; it's my grandson."
>
> THERAPIST: And how did you feel about that?
>
> Ms. Y: I'm hurt and furious. I know it seems really mean, but you don't know how she treats us, ignoring us when we come over and refusing to respond to our calls.
>
> THERAPIST: Well, it sounds like she's behaving in a really hurtful way. But it sounds like your nephew may be the one to pay the price.
>
> Ms. Y: I don't want that to happen. But I really want nothing to do with her. And I'm mad at my brother and mother for just yielding to her.
>
> THERAPIST: This sounds like you're back in the situation with your father, but you're seeing your sister-in-law as acting like him, as her actions seem bullying and controlling. And I think you feel betrayed because instead of forming an alliance against her, like you did with your father, they're not siding with you.
>
> Ms. Y: Yes, I can't believe they won't take my side. I'm so disappointed.
>
> THERAPIST: Yet you know your mother wants to have a relationship with her grandson. I know you feel mad that you can't get them to accept your viewpoint. But the situation is not quite the same as it was with your father. Your sister-in-law is not in control of the family.
>
> Ms. Y: It sure feels like she is.
>
> THERAPIST: I think it's important to recognize how you're caught up in this, because you keep trying to change their behavior. That results in you continuing to feel disappointed and frustrated.
>
> Ms. Y: That's true.

In this instance the patient is perceiving her current circumstance as if she were back in her early life with her tyrannical father. Her sister-in-law had come to represent her father, toward whom she experienced intense hurt, fear, and rage. However, her distress was added to by the disruption of the alliance with her mother and brother. The psychodynamic formulation communicated to the patient helped her to recognize these links. However, in part because of the pervasiveness of her adverse developmental experiences, it would take extensive working through to help her step back and realize she would misread a variety of situations as being traumatic.

References

American Psychiatric Association: Diagnostic and Statistical Manual of Mental Disorders, 5th Edition. Arlington, VA, American Psychiatric Association, 2013

Busch FN: A Model for Integrating Actual Neurotic or Unrepresented States and Symbolized Aspects of Intrapsychic Conflict. Psychoanal Q 86(1):75–108, 2017 28272818

Busch FN, Milrod BL, Singer M, Aronson A: Panic-Focused Psychodynamic Psycho-
    therapy, eXtended Range. New York, Routledge, 2012

Casey PR, Strain JJ (eds): Trauma and Stressor-Related Disorders. Washington, DC,
    American Psychiatric Publishing, 2016

Corradi RB: The repetition compulsion in psychodynamic psychotherapy. J Am Acad
    Psychoanal Dyn Psychiatry 37(3):477–500, 2009 19764847

Freud A: The Ego and the Mechanisms of Defense. New York, International Universities
    Press, 1936

Freud S: Beyond the pleasure principle (1920), in The Standard Edition of the Complete
    Psychological Works of Sigmund Freud, Vol 18. Translated by Strachey J. London,
    Hogarth, 1955, pp 1–64

Kessler RC, McLaughlin KA, Green JG, et al: Childhood adversities and adult psychopa-
    thology in the WHO World Mental Health Surveys. Br J Psychiatry 197(5):378–
    385, 2010 21037215

7

Addressing Personality Disorders

As noted in Chapter 1, personality problems typically include elements from more than a single disorder as classified in DSM-5 (American Psychiatric Association 2013), and therapist and patient work to define components of personality problems that will be addressed. Personality difficulties are approached with the framework described in Chapter 5, with attention to patients' lack of awareness and sometimes aversion to recognizing them. The dynamics will overlap to some extent with those contributing to other problems, such as symptoms and behavioral issues, so that addressing personality factors will aid in relieving these difficulties. This chapter is not a comprehensive review; rather, it is intended to give a sense of the approach to major personality disorders, focusing on Clusters C (characterized by anxious or fearful thinking and behavior) and B (characterized by emotional or unpredictable thinking or behavior and interactions with others) (American Psychiatric Association 2013).

Dependent and Avoidant Personality Disorders

Dependent personality disorder as defined in DSM-5 (American Psychiatric Association 2013) includes the criteria "needs others to assume responsibility for most major areas of his or her life" and "has difficulty expressing disagreement with others because of fear of loss of support or approval" (p. 675). Thus, self and other representations include the notion that one is unable to function effectively alone, often at odds with the patient's actual capabilities, and depends on others viewed as stronger for safety or self-esteem. Patients frequently feel inadequate and humiliated based on their perceived helplessness. Underlying conflicts include a fear that anger will lead to disruption of relationships with significant attachment figures on whom the patient feels dependent. These angry feelings, which may be consciously denied, can trigger anxiety or panic attacks because of this threat, or become self-directed, leading to guilt and self-criticism. Presentation of oneself as dependent or helpless can also help to reassure the patient and others that anger is not a threat. Mentalization is often impaired by attachment fears and the need to view others as strong and in control.

Dependency is frequently associated with idealizing others to allow for a feeling of protection and safety. These idealized representations, however, heighten the fantasy that the other person is necessary for self-esteem or safety. The perception of an idealized other affects the patient's realistic self-assessment, as the self is devalued in comparison to a powerful other, heightening feelings of inadequacy. Disappointments with the idealized attachment figure often occur, triggering conflicted anger. Identifying the tendency toward idealizing others can help the patient to develop a more realistic perception of the capabilities of self and others, helping to diminish feelings of inadequacy and reduce recurrent disappointments.

In targeting dependent personality problems, therapists explore dependent feelings and fantasies, including the contexts that exacerbate them. The therapist helps patients to confront fantasies of their own inadequacy and fragility in comparison to their actual capabilities and to differentiate areas in which they do require support from those which they do not. The therapist aids patients in understanding why they may experience dependent fantasies as humiliating and in easing self-criticism about these wishes. Reduced conflict about these fantasies decreases the threat associated with dependency, diminishes fears of anger, and allows for experimentation with more assertive behaviors.

Case Example

Ms. U, the 45-year-old woman discussed in Chapter 5, suffered from panic disorder, major depressive disorder, and dependent personality disorder. She reported long-standing feelings of helplessness and an inability to manage without others, particularly her husband John. Although she was able to work, Ms. U had struggled with various jobs, believing that her bosses treated her unfairly and did not give her adequate credit. She made a decision with John to quit her job and pursue unfulfilled acting interests. However, after she stopped working, she suffered from an exacerbation of symptoms of depression and anxiety. She was preoccupied about the idea that John could die and was worried about their financial situation, as her husband managed their money. She was fearful that she could not handle things on her own, including financially, because she did not feel safe about returning to work. In addition, she believed that her husband was angry about her requests for money, despite his having supported her quitting, because he would become testy when she asked for funds for her projects. She was anxious and frustrated that he would respond to her requests with a facial expression of displeasure. She feared that she was becoming an increasing burden on him because of her neediness and that he would abandon her.

Ms. U's dependency struggles derived in part from early traumatic experiences with her mother. Ms. U felt abandoned and rejected when her mother drank heavily. She feared her mother would severely injure herself or possibly the patient when intoxicated, leaving Ms. U on her own; her father was emotionally distant and had little involvement with the patient. She reported that her mother was physically and emotionally abusive during her early years, especially when drunk, berating the patient for being "needy" and "fat," even though she was at most mildly overweight. As noted previously, she was deeply conflicted and frightened by her rage at her mother and others; her perceptions of herself as weak and helpless in part helped her to avert her fears. The therapist explored her sense of dependency and the dangers she felt with her husband that had intensified around financial matters:

> THERAPIST: So have you spoken to him about his attitude when you ask for money?
>
> Ms. U: No. He's already in a bad mood about it. If I push him he might blow up and maybe leave.
>
> THERAPIST: Has he ever done this before?
>
> Ms. U: No but you can never tell. I'm also worried he might have a heart attack. He's had some heart problems and he's under a lot of stress from work.
>
> THERAPIST: Well, that's a pretty severe impact just from your bringing up your frustration about his response to your requests for money. You must see your anger as very damaging.
>
> Ms. U: I'm just really worried because I really need him. I'm helpless without him.
>
> THERAPIST: In what way do you feel helpless?
>
> Ms. U: Well, I'm not the one who manages our finances; I depend on him to do that. And I'm worried I won't have enough money.
>
> THERAPIST: I'm not sure that's accurate as we know you can fairly readily find a job as an administrator. I think most of this is transferred from your experience with your mother when you feared she would abandon or attack you or possibly get severely injured or die from her drinking. I think you imagine that your husband would become enraged or incapacitated just as she did.
>
> Ms. U: It's true, he really doesn't tend to respond the way my mother did. I guess I could try talking to him.

Around the same time Ms. U noted a recurrence of certain panic symptoms, including a sensation of unsteadiness, with the associated fantasy that there was nothing to hold onto and she would fall. The therapist asked what came to mind about her symptoms.

> Ms. U: I've been getting palpitations and feeling dizzy. I know I've been stressed, worrying John would leave me, but I also realize I feel furious with him for not supporting me more. Like he doesn't care.

THERAPIST: It's notable that these panic symptoms came back at this
   time. Do you experience them when you get mad at John?
Ms. U: I'll pay attention to that. I think it does tend to happen then.
THERAPIST: What gives you the sense that he doesn't care about you?
Ms. U: I ask him for reassurance that he won't leave me. He says he
   wouldn't leave, but he seems irritated.
THERAPIST: I know you've said he's not very good at expressing emotions or affection. But I wonder if it upsets him that you would
   even think he would leave.
Ms. U: Well, I'm trying to talk to him more about what I feel, but his
   responses are really hurtful. (*Patient is tearful.*) And I guess I get
   furious as well.
THERAPIST: I think that you become frightened of your anger and that's
   adding to your symptoms and fears. You feel unsupported,
   trapped with your feelings and worried about losing control, like
   you felt with your mother. You experience this in your body as
   unsteadiness and dizziness, physical manifestations of feeling
   unsafe and out of control.
Ms. U: Yeah, I'm worried I'll start screaming at him and that will it end
   it for sure. I do experience it in my body. He says he just doesn't
   know how to make me feel better. I know he feels badly sometimes about it.
THERAPIST: I think you're better able to manage on your own and your
   relationship is safer than you imagine.
Ms. U: I already feel less anxious. But I also feel that you're just getting
   tired of this or that you're mad that I'm getting panic again. I feel
   like I'm a burden to you.
THERAPIST: You believe neither me or your husband can tolerate your
   feelings because they are toxic, but you're aware I haven't withdrawn or become angry with you.
Ms. U: No, you're right and I recognize that. It's helpful.

The therapist first worked with her to recognize that she was likely over-
reading the dangers with her husband, including his anticipated abandonment,
adding to her anxiety and sense of helplessness. Ms. U considered the notion
that she was more capable than she gave herself credit for. Identifying her conflicted rage that contributed to her dependency fantasies also aided in her understanding of her panic attacks. As noted at the end of the session, the fears of
abandonment emerged with the therapist, where they could be explored more
directly in the transference.

Patients with avoidant personality disorder are described in DSM-5 as having "feelings of inadequacy, and hypersensitivity to negative evaluation" (American Psychiatric Association 2013, p. 672), and such patients tend to avoid
social situations because they trigger these feelings. Thus, patients tend to view
themselves negatively or as damaged and others as dismissive or rejecting. As
with patients with dependent personality disorder, their dynamics include fears
of expressing anger or self-assertion due to anticipated rejection or criticism,

potentially redirecting anger toward the self. With these patients it is useful to explore situations they are avoiding and to identify the associated negative fantasies contributing to feelings of inadequacy and expected negative judgments. Therapists examine developmental or traumatic factors that have contributed to patients' negative self-evaluation and anticipation of rejection. As their fears are addressed, patients will often attempt to confront situations that they have avoided, providing an opportunity to directly assess fantasized feared outcomes. Mr. P, whose case was discussed in Chapter 4, presented with significant avoidance of social activities.

Obsessive-Compulsive Personality Disorder

Traits of obsessive-compulsive personality disorder include a preoccupation with details, "perfectionism that interferes with task completion," excessive involvement with work, and inflexibility "about matters of morality, ethics, or values" (American Psychiatric Association 2013, p. 678). These patients are often highly self-critical about their inability to meet self-expectations. Rigidity about morality and ethics suggests a severe superego that can lead to depression or low self-esteem. Perfectionism can represent an effort to respond to the demands of a severe superego and a defense against painful feelings of inadequacy. However, perfectionism typically contributes to low self-esteem and anxiety, as patients feel pressured to meet unreasonable goals and expectations. A preoccupation with work and details can function as a defense that allows the patient to avoid the experience of more intense or painful feelings.

The therapist seeks to identify triggers of self-criticism and guilt and aid patients in reevaluating these perceptions. The therapist works to elaborate the content of perfectionistic pressures and help patients recognize and reconsider excessively high self-expectations. Perfectionism and overwork are also explored as unconscious defensive strategies to address underlying feelings of inadequacy and other negative emotions. The therapist will interpret these defenses alongside associated dynamics, such as fears of rejection for not meeting the expectations of others or conflicted rage directed inward via harsh self-attacks.

Case Example

Mr. Z, a 30-year-old lawyer, presented with an intense focus on his work to the exclusion of other activities and interpersonal commitments. He was worried that he was on the verge of a significant professional failure that would cause him to be exposed as incompetent or an impostor. These fears consumed him despite his movement forward on a partnership track at his firm. He also pressured himself to do significant pro bono work which he felt would burnish his reputation at the firm. However, he castigated himself that his work was not "selfless" because he was aware he was deriving personal gain from it.

In reviewing these problems, the therapist and he noted he had a recurrent pattern of fears of failure. He was preoccupied that he would do poorly in law school and not be able to obtain a high-quality job. But after he excelled (including being on law review) and obtained a job at a highly rated firm, he began to worry about passing the bar. He deeply feared that he would fail and would be revealed to be "dumb" relative to his colleagues. He immersed himself in studying for several months and passed easily. Instead of focusing on this accomplishment, Mr. Z then became very self-critical about having been a "bad friend" because he had withdrawn from others to focus on studying for the bar. Subsequently he became preoccupied about performing inadequately at his job at a major law firm. When the therapist asked him if he could take any credit for having obtained this job, he replied, "What would be the point if I fail and get fired?" The therapist noted how themes of extremely high self-expectations and fears of failure underlay this series of difficulties, and it was important to explore where these feelings came from.

Mr. Z reported that his problems had developed following early academic difficulties. He attended an elite private school from age 3 and struggled with reading and writing in his early years. His parents traveled widely and had little interest in his academic struggles. He viewed himself as inadequate relative to his friends and in high school felt "not cool" and unsophisticated compared with his classmates. Somehow over time he was able to develop improved academic skills and performed much better in college. He was furious at his parents for what he viewed as "neglect" of his academic difficulties and their focus on their own interests to the exclusion of his needs.

In the following vignette the therapist addressed his current preoccupation that his pro bono efforts were inadequate:

> MR. Z: So I heard about an associate at our firm who had a very successful pro bono initiative. I've been helping another lawyer provide part time pro bono support for people being evicted from apartments, but now this other lawyer started up his efforts, which have gotten attention from the press. I'm worried that he'll be seen as more successful than I am. And I feel I'm supposed to be doing this work to be selfless, not compete against others. I feel guilty about that.
>
> THERAPIST: It seems like one thing that's consistent in what you describe is a fear of failing to meet expectations. And these expectations are very high and almost impossible to meet. You're both critical of yourself for not doing adequate volunteer work and critical of yourself for not being selfless. You seem to be setting the bar for standards that are impossible to meet, and then when you do meet them you just go on to the next worry.
>
> MR. Z: Well, I know I'm self-critical, but I didn't realize how constant these thoughts were.
>
> THERAPIST: You don't have any graded assessment system. It's all or none.

Mr. Z: That's interesting about the all or none. I've never really thought about it that way. Maybe that could help me with this pressure I feel to work all the time.

The therapist and Mr. Z also focused on his rage at his parents:

Mr. Z: I know we've talked about my disappointment and anger at my parents, but it's been really bugging me lately. Thanksgiving is coming up in a few weeks. When I asked them about it, they said they weren't sure they would be back from a trip then.

Therapist: So it seems like the problems with them haven't changed.

Mr. Z: No, and it reminds me of all the times I needed help that they weren't available.

Therapist: It's important we work on your anger as I think it often gets directed toward yourself. On some level you fantasize that if you're perfect you'll get the attention you desire from your parents and when you're unable to meet these goals you blame yourself.

Mr. Z: I suppose that could be true, but right now I agree we need to focus on my anger, because it's really distracting me from what I need to do.

Narcissistic and Borderline Personality Disorders

Narcissistic and borderline personality disorders are associated with several problems, including mood disorders and recurrent disruptions of close relationships. Targeted psychodynamic treatment approaches have been developed for these disorders (Caligor et al. 2018), particularly borderline personality disorder (Bateman and Fonagy 2016; Yeomans et al. 2015). According to DSM-5, narcissistic personality disorder is characterized by patients' viewing themselves as superior, often exaggerating their achievements, along with expectations that others recognize and admire their talents. They may be preoccupied with fantasies about success and power. Patients typically have a sense of entitlement and expect special favors or treatment from others. The disorder can be accompanied by an inability or unwillingness to recognize the needs and feelings of others. Patients are often envious of others and believe others envy them.

Although DSM-5 emphasizes feelings of superiority or entitlement in these patients, from a psychodynamic standpoint these symptoms are frequently compensatory for feelings of low self-esteem, which are often out of awareness. Their feelings of inadequacy are heightened by disappointments in expectations of responsiveness and admiration. Rather than recognize their injured self-esteem, they become enraged at and devaluing of people who do not recognize their importance. Frequent anger toward and limited empathy with others often disrupt their close relationships. Some patients with narcissistic personality disorder require concrete representations, such as material objects, as evidence of their self-worth and can become depressed and angry when they do not obtain these items.

A key issue in treating such patients is that they usually do not recognize their narcissistic tendencies. They typically respond angrily if someone points out their excessive expectations or entitlement. To engage these patients in treatment, the therapist can explore the circumstances in which the patients feel disappointed in, as well as enraged with, others for not adequately recognizing their capabilities or responding to their demands. Therapists help patients to identify and acknowledge their underlying narcissistic vulnerability and their efforts to manage their self-esteem through compensatory idealized self-views and expectations of others.

Case Example

Mr. AA, a highly successful lawyer, decided to leave his law practice to join a startup developing a legal services software program. However, this new line of work proved to become disappointing and frustrating for him. He was angry with the founders of the firm for not giving him adequate credit for his legal knowledge nor providing him a role that was commensurate with his view of his capacities. Clashes erupted as he demanded more executive tasks and more money. He was told that although his knowledge was important, he did not have adequate technical skills to play the role he hoped for. He decided to leave the company with a plan to return to his old firm, but unexpectedly, at least from his perspective, the firm was not interested. At this point he became severely depressed and sought treatment. His symptoms partially responded to a trial of venlafaxine as the therapist explored his reactions to his circumstances.

> Mr. AA: I didn't realize that the founders of the firm were such idiots. Their plan turned out to be pie in the sky, and the firm is still struggling. If they had listened to my practical advice, they would already have a product worth selling.
>
> Therapist: I realize their behavior was terribly disappointing to you, and it was even more shocking when your old firm did not want you back.
>
> Mr. AA: Well, that's what's really stupid. You would think they would realize how much money they would make from me like they did before.
>
> Therapist: Do you have any idea what happened?
>
> Mr. AA: Well, I'm surrounded by idiots who don't think practically and who don't know how to pursue a business opportunity. But now I feel like such an idiot. I misjudged other people's capacities and look where it's landed me. Now I think no other firm is going to be interested in me. I'm damaged goods.

Rather than his typical railing against others, Mr. AA began to reveal his view of himself as a failure. He had not applied for other jobs, feeling the roles would be beneath him. He believed he would end up at a second-rate firm and lose the respect of others in his area of expertise, but he also feared he might be rejected by other firms. He had dreams in which he was excluded from meetings of his old law partners and felt lost and alone. He believed it was unfair that this had happened to him, and thought this outcome was due to others' lack of recognition or jealousy of his talents.

While Mr. AA's developmental history was being explored, it emerged that both his parents were highly judgmental and critical of him. His father pressured him to excel in competitive sports, often complaining that he wasn't trying his best. From early on he feared that he could not satisfy his mother's academic expectations, and over the course of therapy he concluded that she may have been depressed. Nevertheless, he did well academically, although this did little to relieve his parents' criticisms. He developed a smugness and arrogance, which increased after his acceptance to a prestigious university and law school. Currently, both parents seemed to lack empathy when it came to the pain surrounding his job loss, as they pressed him to "stop messing around and find work."

> THERAPIST: It does seem as if your parents have always judged you critically. It's no wonder that your academic and job success became so important to you.
>
> Mr. AA: My performance in sports was embarrassing to me and my father. It seemed like my skills were finally being recognized when people realized I was smart, though it was still not enough for my mother. Now I'm back to being with idiots.
>
> THERAPIST: I'm wondering whether the people at your startup and firm remind you of your parents, not feeling your talents are enough, and this increases the disappointment and hurt you've felt when they criticize you.
>
> MR. AA: Hmm....Those feelings might be connected. These firms really don't understand my wealth of talents, just like my parents, and they're going to suffer for that.

Here the therapist has allied with Mr. AA in looking at his underlying narcissistic vulnerability and his anger. He also began to work with Mr. AA on his refusal to consider a "second-rate" firm as his unemployment was another problem adding to his depression. He eventually obtained a new job, although he demeaned it. The therapist made efforts to address Mr. AA's behavior of alienating others with his arrogance or unrealistic expectations as problems emerged in his new firm, where he believed the work and people were inferior. The therapist tactfully introduced the idea that his anger with others, as well as how he expressed it could alienate them.

> MR. AA: So the people in this work group are just not good. I made suggestions to them that were very valuable and they rejected them, asking me to come up with a different plan. I told the leader of the group I'm not going to work with idiots.
>
> THERAPIST: And how did he respond?
>
> MR. AA: Not well. He said that they would have to think about reevaluating my contract. But I don't think they will. I'm too successful at what I do.

THERAPIST: We've talked about how hurt and angry you feel when you perceive others don't recognize or "get" you. But perhaps because you feel so strongly sometimes it can be difficult to step back and consider how best to express your feelings. Your responses can hurt and anger others.

MR. AA: I guess I realize that on some level. But I can't stand working with these people.

At this point the therapist explored with Mr. AA what felt intolerable in these circumstances, with some movement in helping him to identify feelings and reactions that added to his negative self-view and interpersonal conflicts. His criticisms of himself and his colleagues diminished. Despite the progress demonstrated in this case, it is important to note that narcissistic personality traits are deeply embedded and can take extended efforts to relieve. Unfortunately many such patients will leave treatment or opt for medication management once their depression has lifted because they tend to feel misunderstood by the therapist (e.g., the therapist does not recognize others are to blame or their entitlement to special treatment) or do not see the value of further exploration of their problems.

DSM-5, in its description of borderline personality disorder as "a pervasive pattern of instability of interpersonal relationships, self-image, and affects, and marked impulsivity" (American Psychiatric Association 2013, p. 663), notes several problems these patients can suffer from. These include abandonment fears, "unstable and intense interpersonal relationships" with "extremes of idealization and devaluation," identity disturbances, impulsivity, suicidality, affective instability with "inappropriate, intense anger or difficulty controlling anger," and "transient, stress-related paranoid ideation or severe dissociative symptoms."

A number of treatments have been developed and tested, including dialectical behavior therapy, transference-focused psychotherapy, and mentalization-based therapy (see Olds and Busch 2014 for a review). Methods and approaches that aid patients in recognizing their distorted perception of others as all good or all bad, managing their rage, and developing mentalization skills are of value. Kernberg's (1967) model of borderline personality disorder delineates the dynamics associated with these problems. Patients are unable to modulate and tolerate negative emotions, such as rage or envy, and they fear, often unconsciously, that they will destroy the needed "good" other, leaving the "bad" other intact. The split perception of others is a defensive reaction to this danger, as rage is directed toward the "bad" other and kept separate from idealized attachment figures. However, the defense of splitting interferes with the development of more complex views of self and others as well as a consolidated identity that can aid in regulation of negative emotions. These idealizations and devaluations are fluid; an "all good" object can suddenly become "all bad." Transference-focused psychotherapy (Yeomans et al. 2015), based on this model, provides an opportunity to address these shifting self and other representations as they emerge with the therapist, helping to clarify and manage the intolerable feelings and defensive splitting.

Problems deriving from these dynamics include poorly managed anger becoming self-directed in the form of severe self-criticism and suicidality. Patients can become depressed or anxious from not having a sense of a secure attachment figure. They can experience recurrent disruptions in relationships related to deficient impulse control and poor management and expression of rage. Helping patients to develop a greater capacity for mentalization (Bateman and Fonagy 2016), to better manage their rage, and to recognize and understand their propensity to split others into all good and all bad can aid in relieving these various difficulties. A broader and more variegated understanding and perception of self and others can help to ease anger, depression, and interpersonal conflicts.

Case Example

Ms. BB, a 48-year-old divorced publicist who presented with periods of severe depression, struggles with intense and unstable relationships, shifting idealization and devaluation of others, bouts of rage, abandonment fears, impulsivity, and suicidality. She felt isolated and frustrated after separation from her husband and recurrent disruptions in relationships with friends, triggered by fights about their not being more helpful to her during her divorce. She had lost interest in her work and had identity struggles concerning what career she should pursue. She was very involved with her family but would feel depressed, angry, and anxious after spending time with them. She would shift from viewing her mother as exploitative, controlling, and help-rejecting, to viewing her as a person who legitimately needed help, a victim of her alcoholic father's harsh criticism and treatment.

When Ms. BB perceived her mother as a victim, she felt guilty about not doing more for her. She felt pressured to "rescue" her mother, but after visiting her parents' home, she became enraged at her mother's unwillingness to listen to the patient or make efforts on her own behalf. Additionally, Ms. BB was criticized by her father, who would refer to her as "mentally ill" and "useless," triggering hurt and rage, followed by a depressed mood and suicidal threats. When enraged at him, she claimed she would not visit home again. In the course of psychotherapy, after multiple unsuccessful medication trials, her treatment was aided by the use of an antipsychotic, quetiapine, and an antidepressant, sertraline, which provided limited easing of her symptoms.

The therapist helped Ms. BB identify a pattern in which she would meet others and initially view their efforts to be responsive to her in a positive way. However, she would subsequently feel disappointed by them, experiencing them as either incompetent, or as having lied to or taken advantage of her. At these points the patient shifted to seeing them as "all bad," viewing them as very hurtful and damaging, and became intensely self-critical for not noticing these problems sooner. When the cycle involving her family restarted and she planned a visit home to help her mother, the therapist attempted to point out these shifting views and how she subsequently felt exploited. She became enraged at the therapist for not understanding her mother or the patient's need to support her, providing an opportunity to explore these factors in the transference.

> Ms. BB: I don't see why you don't get it. My mother desperately needs my help. I have to visit her.
>
> THERAPIST: Yes, but previously after these visits you become very depressed and frustrated with her.
>
> Ms. BB: Well, that's because my father attacks me. He's a total jerk and he keeps her down.
>
> THERAPIST: I understand your feelings about him, but you also get frustrated and disappointed with your mother. Then you become furious with yourself, leading to your feeling depressed.
>
> Ms. BB: I forgot about that. But I have to go there. Right now I just feel guilty I don't spend enough time with her.

In a subsequent session the therapist worked with identifying the shift in her feelings toward him when gripped by her guilt about her mother.

> Ms. BB: I really think I should quit treatment when you talk about reconsidering going home.
>
> THERAPIST: Well, I wonder if the same process goes on here as with your friends. You can find me very helpful, but then you become disappointed when I don't seem to understand you and you become furious with me.
>
> Ms. BB: I know we've discussed this pattern, but right now I think you just don't get it and I'm not sure I see the point in continuing.
>
> THERAPIST: I understand that, but events like this represent a chance to see that angry feelings can be dealt with in a different way from how your family handles them.
>
> Ms. BB: Well right now I'm not finding you too helpful. But I know you have been.

In between these stormy periods Ms. BB became more agreeable about looking at the way her feelings shifted, including in the transference. The therapist worked to identify her pattern of idealization and devaluation of others, her anger and disappointment, and her subsequent self-criticism. Over time she came to recognize how her harshly negative view of others could end up being turned toward herself. She began to consider her own contribution to conflicts with others, and her fears of her own anger being damaging. Another valuable tool for Ms. BB was mentalization, as she began to consider what others might be struggling with internally.

> Ms. BB: I know I shouldn't have gone home but I did do better dealing with my father this time. I was thinking of the things we talked about in his history.
>
> THERAPIST: How did that help?
>
> Ms. BB: I realize he had to deal with his father suiciding. He grew up with just his mother, who was often depressed and drinking. I think

he's very angry and frightened about my mother having problems and worried I might make things worse. This doesn't excuse his behavior, but I understand it better.

These observations led her to form a more complex view of others rather than as all good or all bad, victims or victimizers. This broader range of self and other representations helped to ease her feelings of hurt and anger, and to identify better ways she might interact with others. Although her mood shifts and polarizations continued, the gradual modulation of these states over time aided in relieving her depression and borderline personality symptoms and improving her relationships.

References

American Psychiatric Association: Diagnostic and Statistical Manual of Mental Disorders, 5th Edition. Arlington, VA, American Psychiatric Association, 2013

Bateman A, Fonagy P: Mentalization-Based Treatment for Personality Disorders. New York, Oxford University Press, 2016

Caligor E, Kernberg OF, Clarkin JF, Yeomans FE: Psychodynamic Therapy for Personality Pathology: Treating Self and Interpersonal Functioning. Washington, DC, American Psychiatric Association Publishing, 2018

Kernberg O: Borderline personality organization. J Am Psychoanal Assoc 15(3):641–685, 1967 4861171

Olds DD, Busch FN: Psychotherapy, in Psychiatry, 3rd Edition. Edited by Cutler J. New York, Oxford University Press, 2014, pp 557–609

Yeomans FE, Clarkin JF, Kernberg OF: Transference-Focused Psychotherapy for Borderline Personality Disorder: A Clinical Guide. Washington, DC, American Psychiatric Publishing, 2015

8

Integrating Dissociated Aspects of Self and Other Representations

A variety of problems can stem from a lack of integration of disparate representations of self and others (Table 8–1), which may be in conflict and/or dissociated (Bromberg 1998). For example, a patient may feel unjustly treated by others and at the same time view himself as being "bad" for having rageful or vengeful fantasies toward those he views as mistreating him. Individuals are often unaware of these split-off states of mind, as noted with Ms. BB (see Chapter 7, borderline personality disorder), who did not recognize her shifts between rage toward and guilt about her family. These dissociated representations typically are not at the level of distinct personality states or identities found in dissociative identity disorders (American Psychiatric Association 2013), yet have a profound impact on the individual's psychology (Schimmenti and Caretti 2016). Therapeutic approaches will be described to help patients identify, tolerate, and integrate these variable representations and their contradictory aspects.

Integrating dissociated self/other representations can aid in relief of a range of problems, including anxiety and depression, as well as behavioral and relationship difficulties. For example, Mr. DD, discussed subsequently in this chapter, felt outraged about not getting the credit or attention he felt entitled to, yet simultaneously viewed himself as undeserving and a "loser." This split had led

---

TABLE 8–1.   Dissociated self/other representations

---

1. Not recognized or integrated

2. Frequently linked to trauma

3. Examples

    A.   Submissiveness to demanding others, while feeling outraged about yielding to these demands

    B.   Intense self-criticism for not meeting self and others' expectations, while believing these demands are excessive

    C.   Yielding to bullying others, yet alternately bullying others

---

to his feeling unworthy to ask for support from others, causing him to feel more neglected and angry, as well as anxious and depressed. Recognizing these dissociated representations aided the patient in more effectively seeking support, thus reducing his anger and depression about others not being adequately responsive.

Dissociated self and other representations typically stem from traumatic experiences or recurrent adverse developmental events (Dutra et al. 2009). A common pattern involves pressures to respond to the needs of controlling or critical parents or caregivers. These individuals believe they must yield to the demands of the parent to avoid attack or rejection, while at the same time, they are enraged at the parent's dominating or dismissive behavior. Such pressure can lead to the development of a "false self" (Winnicott 1960), submitting to others' expectations, alongside an aspect of the self that rebels against the demands of others, either directly or through passive aggressive means. These distinct self and other representations are often split off from conscious awareness; patients are frequently surprised by the adverse impact that their angry, rebellious behavior has on relationships, as they view themselves as typically yielding to others. Patients may feel initially justified in expressing their anger, but subsequently may feel terribly guilty, often in an alternating pattern.

These individuals may also develop a view of themselves as "bad," deriving from a perceived failure to meet the parent's expectations and anger at the parent which becomes self-directed. They often feel pressure to monitor and respond to others' needs or distress in an attempt to manage them, maintain control, or prevent rejection. Effective expressions of needs and frustration are made more difficult by dissociated self/other representations, as negative self-views interfere with secure assertiveness. Typically, mentalization is impaired, adding to expectations that others will respond or react in a hurtful or critical manner.

Despite being dissociated, the dynamics, emotions, and behaviors of these disparate representations of self and others greatly influence one another. For example, Mr. DD's sense that he was not worthy of others' attention and the associated pattern of submissiveness contributed to his subsequent rage toward those who failed to recognize his needs and achievements. At the same time, his fear and guilt about his rage further triggered his need to submit and fear of assertiveness. Integration of these representations contributes to the relief of these vicious cycles and more effective emotional regulation.

Recognizing Dissociated Self/Other Representations

Therapists work with patients to identify and integrate split-off self and other representations (Table 8–2). The initial phase of this effort involves bringing these aspects to the patient's attention as they emerge in a variety of circumstances. Once these self/other representations are recognized, the therapist can link them to relevant developmental experiences, helping the patient to understand how they emerged. As this process unfolds, the therapist is alert to and addresses factors that interfere with this recognition. Identifying split-off aspects of self/other representations may create anxiety, pain, guilt, and frustration.

For example, patients may at times fear asserting themselves and in other situations be demanding and bullying. This type of split is not unusual as a consequence of developmental trauma in which patients experienced demeaning or controlling behavior from caregivers. It can be shameful for patients to acknowledge that they are sometimes bullying or controlling when they are frustrated, a form of identification with the aggressor (Freud 1936). The therapist helps patients tolerate and integrate these conflicting aspects of themselves.

Case Example

Mr. I (see Chapters 2 and 6) struggled with dissociated representations of himself and others. The therapist and he identified that in certain situations Mr. I was willing to go out of his way for others and worried about asserting his wishes because he feared being rejected or incurring their wrath. At other times, he became enraged at others for taking advantage of him and not recognizing his efforts or his needs. Occasionally, he would lose his temper and accuse them of exploiting him, which was then followed by intense guilt and self-criticism.

The therapist and patient were able to anchor these representations in the impact of his father's bullying and judgmental behavior. Mr. I felt an intense need to please his father, for fear of being rejected, criticized, or punished. He felt he could not be his true self as his father became demeaning of him or overrode his wishes. For instance, he was interested in attending a drama camp, but his father forced him to go to a camp that emphasized outdoor skills and activities, saying that he needed to "become a man." The therapist explored how these adverse developmental experiences were currently affecting him and worked on integrating the patient's split-off representations, enabling a gradient of response to others' behavior. The patient struggled with these issues, for example, with his girlfriend.

TABLE 8–2.   **Addressing dissociated self/other representations**

---

1. Recognizing dissociated self/other representations

2. Identifying dissociated representations as modes of thoughts, feelings, and behavior

3. Promoting development of agency

4. Engaging in cross talk

5. Effecting integration and mourning

6. Working in the transference

> MR. I: I do so much for her, and I feel she just takes advantage of me. She got mad about the restaurant we went to; she thought it wasn't fancy enough. And then she attacked me for not introducing her to my kids! How can I do that? I hardly have time to spend with them myself.
>
> THERAPIST: So how did you handle that with her? Did you say anything about your frustration with her pressuring you?
>
> MR. I: No. It doesn't do any good. She just gets angrier in response. I'm beginning to feel like I'm being abused by her all the time. And she keeps bringing up things I've done in the past that she thinks were wrong. Like when I asked for advice from a friend who is in fashion about some new suits I was going to get, she said, "Why didn't you ask me? I know about fashion."
>
> THERAPIST: Well, that's a real problem. We know it's not good for you to be in a relationship where you can't speak your mind. But it does feel like a pattern that we've talked about with others and that you experienced with your father. You're fearful of raising your wishes or frustrations because you worry others will attack you. And you feel like you have to do extra for them to ward that off. And then you become angry about feeling taken advantage of.
>
> MR. I: Well, it is kind of like that. When I would say what I wanted the family to do as a kid my father would say, "You don't know anything about this. Shut your mouth!"
>
> THERAPIST: It's almost as if you're repeating the problems in this relationship.

At a later point the patient reported losing his temper with his girlfriend. And notably, he did not connect it with the fearfulness he experienced with her at other times, which the therapist pointed out:

> MR. I: I lost it. I just couldn't take it from her, all these insults. It's too much. I said, "I've had enough of your complaints. Shut up already."
>
> THERAPIST: How did she respond?

MR. I: Oh she was really upset. But the insults just got to be too much. I was furious.

THERAPIST: What do you think happened to your fear that you would wreck the relationship if you said anything?

MR. I: You know I just didn't even think about it.

THERAPIST: Well, it's important to be aware that this can happen to you. Most of the time you're frightened to raise any concerns whatsoever and here you completely lose your temper.

MR. I: It's weird. But she doesn't really get it. She doesn't recognize what she does. I feel I have to talk to her about how she's treated me. Otherwise I just get bottled up. And it shows up in my body. I get terrible headaches. And then I explode.

THERAPIST: You seem to be either overly fearful or explosive. I think we should try to have more of a back and forth between these two sides of yourself. If we think about what it's like when you're furious perhaps we can help you feel safer expressing some degree of anger.

MR. I: That's a good idea, because I need to talk with her about these problems more calmly and not in a rage. But it's hard to do.

The therapist explored with Mr. I how he might shift his behavior to help him feel safer expressing the side of himself that was furious. This approach was discussed in Chapter 5:

THERAPIST: Well, what might you say to her?

MR. I: I might say, "I don't think you realize how completely negative you get toward me. You focus entirely on what I did wrong and you don't even think about all the positive things I've done for you." But I'm really scared about how that's going to go.

THERAPIST: What are you scared of?

MR. I: Well, I think she's going to be really hurt or angry. Maybe she'll stomp off and say she's done with me.

THERAPIST: I think you fear that any expression of your wishes is going to emulate your father's controlling or hurtful behavior toward others. And then when you get enraged you actually behave like he did without realizing it. It's important for you to find a way to express your concerns and frustrations in a relationship without feeling you're going to damage the other person or they're going to reject you.

MR. I: I do have to try to connect with that side of me where I could feel safe getting mad. Maybe that will help me control it better because it just creates problems and I feel guilty. I've never wanted to be like my Dad.

Mr. I was increasingly able to assert his frustration with his girlfriend in an appropriate manner, but she remained highly critical of him. Eventually he ended the relationship. He increasingly grasped how his self and other representations of being bullied or bullying were split off and were connected to his experiences with his father. He became more able to acknowledge that he wanted to bully and control others as he was bullied and controlled. His capacity to develop a more regulated management of his anger in relationships aided in looking for a new partner with whom he could better communicate.

Identifying Dissociated Representations as Modes of Thoughts, Feelings, and Behavior

Another approach to patients with dissociated self/other representations is to identify how their representations are split into different modes of thoughts, feelings, and behaviors, which can be referred to as, for example, mode A and mode B. The therapist can then introduce the concept of a third mode, a mode C, through which there can be an integration of these dissociated aspects.

Case Example

Ms. CC was a 52-year-old divorced mother of two, working as an administrator, who presented with long-standing problems with anxiety and irritability, and the propensity to get into recurrent fights with others. She struggled financially, partly related to difficulties with shopping impulses. She would drink excessively after having a distressing conflict with her family or boyfriend. Her symptoms included several traits of borderline personality disorder (American Psychiatric Association 2013), though her symptoms did not meet full criteria. She described intense pressure to respond to the demands of her family, particularly her father's. Indeed, her father, who still provided financial support, had sent a list of expectations regarding her behavior if he were to continue helping her financially. The list included the instruction that she break up with her current boyfriend, whom the father maintained was "destructive" for her. However, when she did assert herself with the family, she would do so in an aggressive manner that would invariably lead to a fight. For example, the patient reported feeling pressure to host a holiday dinner:

> Ms. CC: I usually do Easter dinner but it's a thankless task. My sister comes and she's very critical and leaves early. She won't do any of the work. I usually don't say anything but this time I said, "Are you going to help me at all and stay longer?" And she said, "You know I'm too busy with work and the kids." And right now I'm fighting with my father, so it will be unpleasant to see him. Plus, I don't like his current girlfriend, who seems to have a problem with me. So this year I think I don't want to do it. I told my sister to screw off, I'm not doing it this year.
> THERAPIST: That may make sense to not host the dinner given what you describe and the tensions you have with the family. But why express it in the way that you did?

Ms. CC: Good question. I mean I just got furious. But then I felt terribly guilty. And alone. Who will I celebrate it with? And I'll feel like I'm like being punished. Now my sister's not speaking with me.

THERAPIST: You seem to experience either one of two modes: one in which you feel unable to resist the pressures of your family and feel guilt ridden, and another in which you get into intense fights with them when you assert yourself. I think we have to understand these different parts inside of you. It seems as though you really struggle with being able to set limits with the family, but then you have terrible battles with them, or do things that are self-destructive, like drinking or shopping.

Ms. CC: Yeah, I see what you're saying about different modes. Most of the time I just automatically yield to what they're saying. And then I get furious and stuck in a bunch of dramatic fights. Now that I'm not going straight to alcohol or shopping, I notice how guilty I feel. It's a similar pattern with my boyfriend.

THERAPIST: It's important to be aware that when you just yield to their demands, you later become furious, and that when you express your anger, you end up feeling terribly guilty. If you can keep both these modes in mind, I think we can help you to be aware that yielding does not work and develop an alternative way of dealing with things. We can think of them as modes A and B and then work to develop a mode C where you can step back from them to take an alternate route.

Ms. CC: Okay, well I can try. I hadn't really thought about what happens with me. Usually I just react.

Promoting Development of Agency

As with Ms. CC, individuals with dissociated self/other representations typically are torn between conflicting aspects of themselves without being aware of it. When these various elements are elaborated, patients sometimes report that they have little control over the conflicting forces they struggle with, just as they felt compelled to either respond to or rebel against the needs of caregivers. It is valuable to address with patients how they do not feel agency over their decisions and may therefore be making choices that are not in their best interest. Integration involves developing a superordinate self (mode C) that helps bring these conflicting factors into awareness to better control their emotions and reduce self-destructive behaviors.

Case Example

Mr. DD, a 45-year-old accountant, had lost his job working for a franchise a year previously and had been unable to find new work. His wife recurrently attacked him about his failure to find a new job, and she "interrogated" him about his daily search efforts. She would also criticize him about his appearance, particularly his being overweight, saying, "You look terrible. You'll never get a job looking like that." They also fought about limit setting with their two adolescent sons. Mr. DD averred that he was unable to stop his wife's attacks, despite his telling her how upsetting they were. The criticisms left him feeling frustrated and powerless, further reducing his motivation to look for a job.

Exploration over the course of treatment revealed four dissociated self/other representations:

1. He saw himself as lazy and being a failure, with intense guilt and an expectation of punishment for not being more motivated in his job search and self-care.
2. He felt furious about the unfairness of his wife's attacks, viewing himself as a victim and wishing others would recognize this mistreatment.
3. He passive-aggressively rebelled by limiting his job search and exercise, exacerbating his wife's and his own sense of himself as a failure.
4. He had a contradictory view of himself as special and expected to be recognized for his talents, almost expecting to be given a job.

The therapist worked to help the patient gain a greater sense of agency over these split-off representations:

MR. DD: So I was talking with this company about a possible job. They want some additional recommendations from prior employers. I gave them one already. They requested this a couple days ago and I've just put it off.

THERAPIST: Why do you think you've put it off?

MR. DD: First it seemed like they were ready to hire me. I'm not sure what happened. I mean I did ask for more money because I felt they would be underpaying me. So I think asking me for more recommendations means that maybe they're not interested anymore.

THERAPIST: That raises a couple of issues. First, it's interesting that you're asking for more money when you really need the job. But I also wonder why you are surprised that they would ask for additional letters of recommendation?

MR. DD: Look, I don't think it's right they would underpay me. Maybe I did drive them away by asking for more money. But I don't think they need more recommendations. I should be a shoo in for this job.

THERAPIST: I see this as part of the patterns we've talked about. You expect that you will be rejected from a job and, simultaneously, that you should just be given a job.

MR. DD: I find it confusing, but I do recognize both those parts. I am mad that they just don't see I'm qualified and are making me jump through hoops. Another thing is that my wife is torturing me about it every minute. "What's happening? Did I get the recommendations?" And you know that saps my motivation further.

THERAPIST: I think we understand that your anger at her contributes further to that slowdown. But there's a lot of factors that keep this behavior from changing. Your anger at not feeling properly recognized, your fear of rejection, your frustration with your wife, and wanting to demonstrate that you're a victim. But one thing connects these areas. You don't seem to be in charge. There's no sense of agency.

MR. DD: I want people to get how unfairly I've been treated. To recognize it and have some sort of sympathy.

THERAPIST: Well, that aspect is important to you, but you've said you would feel better if you got a job, and it's financially necessary! But you get caught up by these various conflicted parts of yourself. I think it would be helpful for you to recognize that finding employment is primary for you, and then try to address the pulls that interfere with your making progress, like to rebel or show you're a victim. We can look at how these other factors get in the way.

MR. DD: You think that will help me get it done? Of course I want a job.

THERAPIST: I think it's definitely worth trying, because I think you get stuck between all these parts of yourself pulling at you.

For Mr. DD, establishing a sense of agency required recognizing how these split-off representations interfered with his judgment, often out of awareness or in a piecemeal fashion. He grew up feeling neglected by his father, who was not responsive to his feelings or interests and was emotionally distant. He felt pressured to try to please his father with academic success and at the same time was enraged at the lack of recognition. His sense of specialness was compensatory for his underlying low self-esteem but left him more vulnerable to frustration and disappointment. These conflicts were mirrored in his current circumstances with his job search and his wife. Gaining an understanding of these factors was essential for his being able to effectively assert himself in both these areas.

Case Example

Mr. N (see Chapter 4) had split representations between a view of himself as a failure and a perception of himself as a rebel, critical of standard conventional lifestyles. The therapist worked with him to recognize these dissociated states, easing his depressive symptoms.

MR. N: I know I was triggered when I went to my sister-in-law's house. I felt really bad about myself and kept thinking about how I haven't accomplished anything like these people have. They have two Porsches. I mean I'm not into cars, but I feel I haven't made the money I need to make to be one of the wealthy people.

THERAPIST: Yes, but even as you say that I know you've been very critical of that lifestyle, that you consider it shallow and ostentatious.

MR. N: Well, I really remember how much I loved the conventional lifestyle, back when I was a kid. I loved the comfortable home and nice TV and my bedroom. I really bought into the whole thing. But then it all completely fell apart. My parents got into these terrible fights and sometimes the cops were called. They split up when I was 11 and then that's when my father's abusive behavior started. Things fell apart for me. And I guess I want them to know this lifestyle isn't real. You think it is but this isn't how people really work. And I'm not really interested in the materialism. I'm interested in books, art, and music.

THERAPIST: So that's something we really need to understand. How can you be so critical of yourself for being a failure with regard to making money when you don't even agree with those aspirations?

MR. N: It's a good question. I'm beginning to see how I'm back and forth about these things.

THERAPIST: I think that your sense of failure stems from taking in your father's view of you. You were enraged at him but couldn't find any way to express it. I think you turned a lot of that anger against yourself.

MR. N: Well maybe that's it. I know I make fun of that lifestyle. I really feel alive when I'm off doing my own thing like hiking. I just don't like when others are ostentatious. I didn't want to be at this family event and see my cousins with their fancy cars. That stuff doesn't speak to me. But I left feeling like a terrible failure. I didn't achieve what they did. I spent all those years working as an art framer. I mean they were prestigious paintings. It was a skill. But I didn't end up with anything from it.

THERAPIST: It's curious how you usually shift to a negative view of yourself and your work. And the healthy part of yourself and this negative view don't communicate with each other. You don't say, "Well, I feel bad I don't have as much money as my cousins, but you know having a fancy car just doesn't appeal to me. I really like playing music." Or, "You know I did develop a skill, art framing, while I tried to pursue my artistic interests. I was able to get paid for it."

MR. N: Yes, it's interesting. It's like I lose sight of that side of me when my self-esteem drops. I plunge into this deep hole.

Engaging in Cross Talk

Once patients recognize disparate self and other representations, integrating them requires significant working through (see Chapter 9). Recognizing dissociated representations often creates conflict and can trigger anxiety or pain. Additionally, these representations have existed preconsciously and reflexively over many years, and therefore take considerable time to integrate and modify. Analogies can be made to learning a new instrument or language; one can learn to recognize notes or words, but it will take considerable practice and repetition to gain skill in these areas. *Cross talk* is a term for an approach that patients can learn to address their split-off self/other representations, using "mode C." Cross talk consists of the patient addressing one part of the self to the other, while recognizing that this effort may create distress or resistance.

Case Example

The therapist talked to Mr. P (see Chapters 4 through 6) about how his feelings of failure were added to by grandiose fantasies that compensated for his feelings of insecurity:

> THERAPIST: I think that you felt deeply insecure and inadequate growing up, and you attempted to deal with that by fantasies of being in charge and defeating your enemies. However, you are recurrently disappointed by your inability to fulfill these wishes and switch back to thinking of yourself as a failure or bad in some way. But these different ways of viewing yourself don't occur at the same time.
>
> MR. P: Well, how do you get one part of yourself to talk to another?
>
> THERAPIST: I think it's important to recognize that you've become more successful and you're no longer that inadequate boy on the verge of getting into trouble.
>
> MR. P: But as you know I'm always worried that a reprimand is coming just around the corner or that I'm going to get fired.
>
> THERAPIST: I think it's important that you challenge these ideas when they arise. If you find yourself thinking you're on the verge of being fired, it's important to remember that you're thought of very highly and that has been reflected by strong reviews and salary increases. You may not be in charge of the company as you hope in your fantasies, but you're doing very well.
>
> MR. P: I see. I don't think challenging these feelings is easy, but I've never really tried that.

Case Example

Mr. F (see Chapter 2) struggled with alternating rage at others for not recognizing his specialness, his expression of those feelings passive aggressively in his unwillingness to complete tasks, and a sense of failure for not accomplishing more. The therapist helped to find ways of integrating these aspects of himself:

> MR. F: I rebel against capricious authorities, and I guess I view my wife in that way. I feel I shouldn't have to do these menial tasks, like cleaning up dishes, and I shouldn't have to get a job. But then part of me fears confrontation with my wife or others who get furious that I don't do these things. At other times I become really self-critical. I think I'm irresponsible.
>
> THERAPIST: These different aspects of yourself don't seem connected with each other. Maybe because it's too dangerous to think of them together.

Mr. F: I see what you're saying, but how would I connect them?

Therapist: You could think, "Well, I'm really furious I have to do these things, but if I don't, I'll have a terrible confrontation about it or end up feeling like a failure or guilty."

Mr. F: I've never really done that. It's very frustrating to be so stuck.

Therapist: It also feels as if you don't have agency to decide things. You're at the mercy of this struggle with authority, and you either yield or rebel.

Mr. F: I think part of the problem was that my parents might have given up on limit setting. They just sort of let me do what I wanted. Like when I didn't do my homework my father did it for me. But I think in the end I'll just be mad even if I do the things I'm supposed to.

The patient became more aware of these split-off representations but found integration difficult. He and the therapist considered creative ways to reach these goals:

Mr. F: I guess I see what you're saying now. These parts of myself seem to run independently. They don't really communicate with each other. Maybe we can try putting them in a room together and have them talk to each other.

Therapist: Okay, let's try that.

Mr. F: I imagine that they don't want to talk to each other because they're all sad and angry. There's the rebellious guy who can't or won't do what he's supposed to. There's the self-critical person who attacks himself for not getting things done. There's the guy who doesn't feel better even when he does the things he's supposed to because nobody recognizes his efforts. And none of them want to talk to each other.

Therapist: So what if we imagine someone more rational who tries to negotiate between them.

Mr. F: I imagine the rational guy tries to broker some kind of compromise but nobody's interested. They're all too angry. One guy is like: What do I get out of this if I give up porn or do the dishes? The other guy is angry and says I won't do it or I can't do it. And the third guy just remains self-critical. So they don't get anywhere.

Therapist: But you already seem to have given up on a positive outcome even though you just identified these parts of yourself.

Mr. F: That's true.

Therapist: And all the negotiation points you imagine are negative. What about the self-critical person being relieved when chores get done or the rebellious guy expressing anger by showing others he can work rather than by refusing to?

Mr. F: It's hard for me to think of it that way but I'll consider it. It's very difficult to deal with things when you have all these people in your head pulling in different directions. I'm worried because they've added some work to my part time job, and now I think that my rebellious side will kick in, the "won't/can't" guy. Because once I think I'm being pushed I get stuck.

Case Example

Mr. J (Chapters 2 and 3) steadily gained ground on understanding his split-off attacks toward himself, which he had previously accepted as making sense and being appropriate. He was increasingly aware of when these occurred and questioned the accuracy of those criticisms. One approach that was useful in this work was exploring the mechanism by which his rage at his mother became internalized in vicious self-attacks. The therapist and Mr. J first identified that these attacks happened after becoming enraged toward his mother. They then determined that this anger became unacceptable for him, either because he could not tolerate viewing his mother as so damaging or because he felt it was wrong for him to be so furious. At that point he accepted his mother's attacks on him and directed his anger toward himself. The therapist also helped Mr. J recognize that the content of his self-criticisms mirrored his mother's attacks on him. Then they worked to tolerate and accept the degree of hurt and rage he felt with his mother.

Working with two dreams aided this process. In the first his mother cut skin on Mr. J's hand and pulled it back. His mother then set it into place with hypodermic needles. Mr. J experienced intense pain and rage toward her. He had never felt so angry and was unsure he could contain it. In the second dream he became furious at his wife. He acknowledged that she hadn't really done anything wrong to him recently but was still as enraged as he had been at his mother.

In associating to the first dream, he recalled many instances in which his mother would attack him unfairly, including calling him "lazy" and "stupid." She seemed particularly incensed when Mr. J garnered interest from girls.

THERAPIST: What would she say to you then?

MR. J: After they came over there was like a barrage of attacks. She would say I was lazy and not doing my homework. She told me that I was making my sister feel bad because boys weren't interested in her because she was overweight. And she would say I was going to get grounded if she found out anything was going on sexually with these girls. In the meantime I hardly knew what she was talking about. We weren't doing anything that terrible when we went out.

THERAPIST: It sounds like she made you feel very badly about some positive things about yourself, including girls being interested in you. We might wonder if she was even competitive with you or the girls.

MR. J: I hadn't thought of it that way. And the needles reminded me of her taking me to the orthodontist. I had a lot of problems with my teeth that required all these procedures. It was so painful. I took needles and shots because the mask to put me to sleep terrified me. And my mother was horrible about it. She just told me to stop making trouble.

THERAPIST: I think in the dream the pain you felt when your skin was pulled back is like the mental pain you experience with her. What about the second dream?

MR. J: There's nothing terrible my wife did recently, but I was talking to my friend about her husband. He's really being abusive toward her. I know I get angry at my wife but she's nothing like this.

THERAPIST: Did the conversation remind you again of your mother?

MR. J: I guess it did. Her husband says a lot of hostile things toward my friend and demeans her, like my mother does with me.

THERAPIST: I think one thing that happened in these dreams is that you got in touch with the full intensity of your rage toward your mother. Maybe that's a breakthrough because if you can safely experience those feelings, it would help you to not turn it on yourself.

MR. J: Yes, but I did start attacking myself yesterday for getting angry at the gym. It's all younger people and they were showing off how much they could lift. I feel like I'm in the way. It's exactly why I didn't want to go to this gym. Then I'm like "what's wrong with me that I can't tolerate anything?"

THERAPIST: I wonder if you started to attack yourself after your friend's story reminded you of your mother. You probably got angry at her and then turned it on yourself.

MR. J: I didn't think of that, but I know that's the pattern. How come I can't recognize these things?

THERAPIST: I think you are increasingly recognizing them, but again you're sounding self-critical. You not only attack yourself for getting mad but when you feel in pain.

MR. J: I do say, "Why are you getting depressed again? What's wrong with you?" I guess I just keep turning these things around on myself.

The session ended with the therapist highlighting how the patient's access to his rage in the dream presented an opportunity to feel safer with it and not immediately attack himself. The patient responded: "If I ever did get mad, she said I was being ungrateful and not appreciating all the wonderful things she did for me. So then I would feel even worse." These experiences provided additional information for therapist and patient to work further on how the patient's anger became immediately self-directed and how to address it.

Effecting Integration and Mourning

Integration often involves the acceptance of painful realities about oneself and one's caregivers. Patients shift to a more complex understanding of self and others, including the stresses their parents experienced, as their mentalization skills increase. Mr. N (See Chapters 3 and 4), for example, was describing distressing early experiences that he remembered after the previous session, including the fear of his father's attacks and feelings of humiliation.

> MR. N: He would give me these quizzes. He was very well read, and I had no idea what the answers were. I was in a rebellious teenage phase. I would just feel humiliated and stupid. And he would say "You'll never amount to anything."
>
> THERAPIST: I believe you internalized these negative self-views and even now attack yourself as a failure, despite the successes you've had in your life.
>
> MR. N: I'm getting better at stopping myself from going to that place. I also recalled my intense social anxiety. I remembered visiting my cousins who were attractive and intelligent, and I so much wanted to impress them. Because they seemed so warm and so different from my family and the abuse I was receiving. I just wanted the attention. I hate admitting that.
>
> THERAPIST: We need to understand what you hate about it because it seemed like you would desperately want the approval and security you weren't getting at home.
>
> MR. N: It was like there was this dark and negative side that my father represented. And yet I've been thinking about what he went through growing up. His mother was like bat-shit crazy: very seductive at times and at other times screaming at him. Also I found out he kept track of my career accomplishments, but I didn't find out until after he died. And that's really sad.
>
> THERAPIST: So there's the realization that he did acknowledge your success but did not tell you directly. He was wrong about your not amounting to anything; maybe he recognized it. Tell me about what's sad.
>
> MR. N: That he behaved so terribly toward me, and it's tragic what he experienced. And he could never openly acknowledge anything positive.
>
> THERAPIST: I think this is part of the ongoing process of integrating these parts of yourself. You recognize the complexity of what you suffered and what your father experienced. It's not that you were a failure, and you've found how people view you in very positive ways you didn't expect.
>
> MR. N: It's important for me to consider that because once I go into those negative self-attacks it's like I'm falling off a cliff.

Working in the Transference

The transference provides another opportunity to identify dissociated self and other representations in relation to the therapist (see Ms. BB in Chapter 7). The therapist addressed this split as it emerged with Mr. I (see Chapters 2 and 6) during a discussion about a fee increase:

> MR. I: I'm angry that you mentioned increasing the fee. It makes me think that you're just mercenary. You only care about the money and not about me.
>
> THERAPIST: It's hard for you to consider the possibility that I can both care about you and be paid because this is my livelihood.

Mr. I: I think other doctors wouldn't raise their fee. I think it shows what your priorities are. And how you're really not concerned about what's best for me.

Therapist: I understand that you see this as not responsive to your needs or uncaring. But I do think you're vulnerable to experiencing others as behaving in ways that are disregarding like with your father growing up.

Mr. I: I see what you're saying, but somehow I want to make it more about you.

Therapist: We can talk more about what you think my motives are, but it can be helpful for you to recognize that you're vulnerable to feeling disregarded and react strongly to it, because sometimes you misperceive others as behaving malevolently. And it adds to your viewing their behavior as only focused on themselves.

Mr. I: Apropos of that story, my father did upset me a lot last night. My son got deferred at his top choice college. And my father contacted me because he felt I needed his advice. He started telling me a series of steps my son should take regarding his college applications. I said that I thought it was important to see what my son wanted to do. And he responded: "Well, I don't want to tell you what to do in this situation." I was so annoyed! I'm a middle-aged adult! I know how to deal with these things.

Therapist: I understand your frustration in that your father says he doesn't want to tell you what to do when that is precisely what he is doing. And he acts as if you're not capable of handling it.

Mr. I: And I get mad and I really want to tell him off, but I'm too frightened to do it.

Therapist: Because you fear he'll retaliate by putting you down. Since he feels he knows best, he doesn't respond well when you express your independent opinion.

Mr. I: No, he doesn't, and when I was a kid, it was really scary to be around him. And I'm still frightened of him.

Therapist: But you do have more perspective. And it's not like you didn't respond. You did say to him that your son should have a role in these decisions.

Mr. I: That's true.

Therapist: You also have the opportunity to look at this in your relationship with me. You worry I'm going to attack and undermine you, yet you were able to express your frustration about the fee. And you see we just talked about it and I didn't attack you for it.

Mr. I: I do see it's different. I hope this allows me to be more direct in other situations. It's scary to give my opinion, but I told you how I felt and it seems to have worked out.

References

American Psychiatric Association: Diagnostic and Statistical Manual of Mental Disorders, 5th Edition. Arlington, VA, American Psychiatric Association, 2013

Bromberg PM: Standing in the Spaces: Essays on Clinical Process, Trauma, and Dissociation. Hillsdale, NJ, Analytic Press, 1998

Dutra L, Bureau JF, Holmes B, et al: Quality of early care and childhood trauma: a prospective study of developmental pathways to dissociation. J Nerv Ment Dis 197(6):383–390, 2009 19525736

Freud A: The Ego and the Mechanisms of Defense. New York, International Universities Press, 1936

Schimmenti A, Caretti V: Linking the overwhelming with the unbearable: developmental trauma, dissociation, and the disconnected self. Psychoanal Psychol 33(1):106–128, 2016

Winnicott DW: Ego distortion in terms of true and false self, in The Maturational Processes and the Facilitating Environment: Studies in the Theory of Emotional Development. London, Karnac Books, 1960, pp 140–152

9

Working Through

As demonstrated in many of the vignettes in this book, problems often have multiple dynamic contributors and serve a variety of functions. Working through (Freud 1914) involves the process of identifying these dynamic factors and how they emerge in different contexts and circumstances (Table 9–1). For instance, patients may be unassertive because of expectations that others will respond to assertive behaviors in a punitive fashion; fears of damaging others or disrupting relationships through self-assertion; and guilt about wishes to harm, control, or humiliate others linked unconsciously with assertive behaviors. Identifying each of these dynamic factors helps patients to feel safer expressing their needs and wishes. Patients can explore how these dynamics operate during and outside of sessions in a variety of contexts, including in the transference, as well as with family, friends, and colleagues. Over the course of treatment, the increasing awareness of the dynamics and contexts surrounding problems provides a range of opportunities and strategies for relieving them.

A key additional step is demonstrating how specific dynamics overlap in contributing to various problems patients struggle with. This technique helps to reinforce and more rapidly address the patient's range of difficulties. For instance, as described in the case of Ms. C (see Chapters 1 through 3 and 5, and below), conflicts about angry feelings viewed as potentially disruptive to relationships can contribute to unassertiveness, panic symptoms, and anger directed inward in the form of self-criticism and associated depression. In working through, patients learn to become more aware of their angry feelings, identify triggers of these feelings, tolerate and accept them, and express anger more appropriately. The impact of changes on these dynamics will often aid in relief of various problems in an interactive and cumulative manner. Improved recognition and tolerance of anger, for example, can help increase assertiveness and reduce anxiety and depression.

TABLE 9–1.   Working through
1.   Recognize that multiple factors and functions contribute to problems
2.   Identify dynamic contributors to difficulties in different contexts
3.   Determine strategies to intervene with problems based on these dynamics
4.   Examine how dynamics overlap in contributing to various difficulties

Finally, working through enables an assessment of how the patient is progressing in managing and easing various problems. With some difficulties there may be significant improvement, whereas in others little change may have occurred. This process can aid in determining how to best focus interventions in addressing persistent problems. As will be noted in Chapter 10, identifying the degree of change can help to determine when termination should be considered.

Identifying Various Contributing Dynamics to Problems

Several different dynamic factors can contribute to the development and persistence of specific problems. Oftentimes a problem will persist until the patient becomes aware of these various contributing dynamics and, with the therapist, determines strategies for addressing them (Table 9–2). Therefore, it is important for the therapist to look for additional relevant dynamics and determine how they interact with those that have been identified.

Case Example

Mr. J (Chapters 2, 3, and 8) described struggles with loneliness, which he recognized would shift to feelings of being rejected and depressive symptoms. He and the therapist determined that for Mr. J, aloneness was linked to childhood experiences of feeling rejected by his mother and, to some extent, excluded by his father, who spent much of his time alone in his office. This connection was reinforced by his parents' punishments of him, which included being sent to his room for hours at a time. Therefore, he associated being alone with being "bad." These feelings were reinforced by constant criticisms by his mother, who said he was "sluggish" and "thoughtless" and had "bad friends."

As therapy progressed, he increasingly recognized how being alone triggered depression and self-attacks. He would then anticipate others being excluding, rejecting, and punitive toward him, and use that information to increase contact with others to relieve his fears. However, he continued to struggle with episodes of intense self-loathing. In this part of the working through process, therapist and patient further explored how his aloneness and anger led to self-attacks, and discussed how he was handling these feelings:

TABLE 9–2. **Approaches to working through**

Identifying various contributing dynamics to problems

Identifying the impact of dynamic factors in varying contexts

Addressing circumstances in which problems persist

Identifying backlash as progress is made

Using transference as an aid to working through

Applying overlapping dynamics to various problems

MR. J: I was feeling really down on Wednesday. I know I was alone too much. I told Susan she was going out too often and needed to be at home more. And I told my friend to come meet me at work for lunch. But I was still really struggling.

THERAPIST: What do you think contributed to that?

MR. J: Well, I've had a series of grants that were rejected. And I start to think it's my fault, although I know that it's not. The government just doesn't have the money for these projects. But then I start in on myself, "You're a failure. You're no good. That's why you didn't get these grants."

THERAPIST: That's what we've seen before. When you feel alone and rejected you start to blame yourself. You must have done something wrong to deserve the punishment you were getting.

MR. J: Yeah, because my mother kept telling me that. And she said I was to blame for my sister having problems even though I didn't have anything to do with it. And then my mother sent me to boarding school because I was supposedly a "bad kid" because girls were interested in me. I was completely alone there. I couldn't tell my parents or teachers that my roommates bullied me. I was miserable and there was no one to talk to about it.

THERAPIST: At the same time you felt, and even now feel, enraged about the unfair treatment you were getting. You were unfairly viewed as causing problems, and some of your positive attributes were seen as creating trouble. But your rage doesn't feel safe, in part because you feel you'll be punished for it by being sent off to be alone.

MR. J: Yes, And now that you mention it, I was getting really infuriated. And I didn't really know how to handle it. Recently, I was furious at one organization for not giving us a grant. I mean they have the money, but they're really tight with it. Even so, I started attacking myself, "If you were better at this then they would have given you the money. You're a failure." But then I went and screamed at Susan for going out too much and then felt horribly guilty. Then I settled down, and she agreed to cancel a couple of plans. She was okay about it. I felt a bit better.

THERAPIST: It seems like in this instance you dealt effectively with your rage. First you attacked yourself with the same criticisms your mother directed toward you. Then you recognized you were feeling alone and self-critical and you used your anger to help find a solution to those feelings.

MR. J: Yes, being alone and struggling with my anger seem to get caught up together.

THERAPIST: So we know it's important to pay attention to feeling both lonely and mad. Because when you were growing up you didn't have any way to express these feelings effectively.

MR. J: Are you kidding? If I started fighting with my mother or criticizing her, it would be way worse. She would send me to my room for hours. But now I'm on the lookout for these feelings so I can avoid attacking myself.

Identifying the Impact of Dynamic Factors in Varying Contexts

In the working-through process, therapists aid patients in identifying how dynamics and developmental factors are relevant to the emergence of a problem in varying contexts. For example, as noted in Chapter 8, patients with histories of traumatic or adverse events often experience certain current circumstances as if the traumatic experience were recurring, typically out of awareness. Being able to identify these perceptions and feelings in various contexts enables patients to recognize how much they are affected by these events and under what circumstances this impact occurs. This examination helps build patients' capacities to step back from and identify how they misread relatively benign situations as traumatic.

Case Example

Mr. N (Chapters 3, 4, and 8) described his ongoing struggles with mistrust of others and depression, as he spoke about how presenting his own views on a variety of issues was affected by the political polarization that he experienced with his friends and family:

MR. N: I'm struggling because I get so upset with people making these statements when they really haven't looked at the facts. I feel the news stations distort the truth. They take political stances rather than just looking at the facts. I actually study the data about these issues. If they involve science, I'll actually read the research papers. But if I try to talk to people about what I read, they get mad at me and don't want to budge from their position. I just feel helpless. And I get preoccupied with it. I can't let it go.

THERAPIST: It seems to mirror how you felt you were lied to as a child and the damage that caused. And how you weren't listened to growing up.

MR. N: I was told that there I was in this wonderful family and every-thing was okay. But then I watched it just deteriorate and col-lapse around me with my parents' violent fights and divorce. I just don't like this deception. Then I start to feel excluded by oth-ers like I'm some kind of a rebel freak when I try to talk to them. Similar to how I felt in high school. I'm hurt that people don't want to listen to me when I have these facts.

THERAPIST: I think that you're caught in your traumatic experience when you perceive and react to things in this way. It's under-standable that you would be furious when facts are distorted, but I think the intensity and preoccupation are added to by your dis-appointment and trauma in childhood. You feel helpless, en-raged, and fearful of feeling excluded as you were as a kid. But it's important to recognize that people feel very intensely about these political issues, and it's less about your ideas. Maybe if you could recognize how polarized people are in their views you could present the information in a manner where they might hear you.

MR. N: That's a good way to look at it. Because people really aren't thinking about these political issues. It's all or none. In business we talk about how to present something in a way that people can hear it. I could do that. I'm feeling better thinking about this now.

THERAPIST: Your business idea also represents a place or stance where you can step back from trauma and experience things differently. I think that's what happened when you calmed down just now. And your ability to recognize what's going on with others from that standpoint reminds me of how you saw your father differ-ently when you recognized the impact of his background on his behavior.

Addressing Circumstances in Which Problems Persist

Often problems will generally resolve but continue to be triggered in certain cir-cumstances. The notion that problems will emerge in some contexts more than others was discussed as an important area of exploration in Chapter 1. Thera-pist and patient can work to apply the knowledge of the dynamics and strategies they have gained to identify and address remaining triggers of difficulties.

Case Example

Ms. EE was a 57-year-old university professor, the oldest of seven children in her family, with a long history of anxiety and depression and a tendency to yield her needs to those of others. She described growing up with a very needy mother who had constant somatic complaints and spent much of her time in bed. The patient had excessive demands placed on her due to her mother's professed inability to manage the children. She was forced to step in for her mother despite it being much more than she could handle. In relationships she felt intense pressure to take care of others and was terrified that she would fail to adequately respond to them. However, she had developed some capacity through treatment to recognize and understand this tendency and intervene before acting on it. The patient described progress in asserting her needs but persistent problems with her mother.

> Ms. EE: My friend had asked me if my dog could stay with her while I went on a trip. She's a therapy dog, and my friend was having a hard time. In my usual manner I said, "Yes. Sure." But then I thought, "Wait, what if I'm anxious about my trip?" I want her to be able to come with me.
>
> THERAPIST: It sounds like your usual reflexive behavior, "I need to take care of the other person's needs." But then you were able to step back and think, "What about my needs?" That's not something you were able to do before.
>
> Ms. EE: Yes, I was encouraged about that. But my mother's been ill, and she's very anxious. She's acting like the mother of my childhood. You know, she's making her usual demands that I come take care of her, and I'm feeling tremendous pressure to do it. The other day I canceled a class to take her to see her doctor. I really shouldn't be doing this kind of thing.
>
> THERAPIST: One thing that's important to understand is that you've developed this capability to step back and observe the pressure you feel to respond to others' needs, but in the case of your mother that ability just disappears. What do you think disrupts your capacity at that point?
>
> Ms. EE: I just don't even think of it sometimes. There's so much pressure and I go into an autopilot mode and acquiesce to her demands.
>
> THERAPIST: You may feel most in danger with her. But maybe you could think about it like with your friend, where the impulse to let her spend time with your dog was followed by remembering to examine that urge.
>
> Ms. EE: I can try to keep that in mind with my mother and see what happens. Maybe I can stop myself from going on autopilot.

Identifying Backlash as Progress Is Made

Patients often experience anxiety and guilt as they move forward with changes in their feelings and behaviors (Freud 1916/1957). These feelings can lead to a form of backlash, including a resurgence of their fears. They may also trigger a type of undoing, characterized by the onset of self-criticism or expectation of attack, including from the therapist, regarding their progress. It is important for the therapist to identify this pattern as it indicates areas of persistent conflict and helps recognize factors interfering with positive changes.

In a subsequent session, Ms. EE described a shift in her awareness of her own needs, which created a threat for her:

> Ms. EE: I had the idea, "Let me come in and talk about myself for a change." And that is different, because normally I just talk about other people's needs.
>
> THERAPIST: That is an interesting shift.
>
> Ms. EE: So I was thinking about this woman I really like; she helps me with paperwork and some chores around the house. And I was wondering what I like so much about her.
>
> THERAPIST: What comes to mind?
>
> Ms. EE: Well, I guess she does things for me. I don't need to worry about doing things for her. Except pay her of course.
>
> THERAPIST: So it's kind of the opposite of what you're used to?
>
> Ms. EE: Yes. I hadn't thought about it that way before, but it's really nice to feel like that. And I noticed I can be silly with her. I like to make jokes. And with her I can do more of it.
>
> THERAPIST: So you feel safe to let go around her.
>
> Ms. EE: Yes, I do. But do you think it's okay to be silly?
>
> THERAPIST: What would be wrong with it?
>
> Ms. EE: Well, I think I'll get into trouble for it.
>
> THERAPIST: Because it's too far from taking care of other people? It's just having fun.
>
> Ms. EE: It's the opposite of where I often feel I need to be. But if I just become silly in here and make some jokes, then I'm sure you would get annoyed and think, "She's not serious about therapy or working through her problems."
>
> THERAPIST: I don't think so. I would see it as a sign of progress and a sign you were feeling safer and able to have more fun.
>
> Ms. EE: Oh, that's surprising to me!

Case Example

Ms. Q (Chapter 4) was able to more directly confront her husband about his problematic behavior. However, she then experienced guilt about her greater assertiveness:

> Ms. Q: I really couldn't take it anymore. I felt like I was losing control, but I told him to get out of the house for the day. He was hurt, but he accepted it. When he returned he was actually less morose and irritable.
>
> THERAPIST: So it seems like you're more willing to try to protect yourself by setting limits on his behavior. You've always concluded that you're a failure or in the wrong, thus you don't deserve or can't get protection.
>
> Ms. Q: Yes, I was surprised that he responded the way he did.
>
> THERAPIST: We know that growing up you felt you had to just accept your father's view of you as bad. And there was nothing you could do about it.

Ms. Q: I guess I've just been used to that helplessness. But my anger
      didn't come out in a good way.
Therapist: What do you mean?
Ms. Q: Well, I feel I was too harsh in the way I expressed it.
Therapist: What was too harsh?
Ms. Q: Well, it's mean to tell him to get out of the house. But I just
      couldn't stand it. And he was being nasty to our son in addition
      to being sullen and withdrawn.
Therapist: People don't always say things nicely when they're angry.
      But I think it would be hard for you to feel comfortable express-
      ing theses wishes in any way. We can work on finding better ways
      to communicate your anger now that you are more aware of it.
      I think you felt a wave of guilt because inside you feel you don't
      have a right to express your needs and in this case you did it very
      strongly. But things did improve afterward.
Ms. Q: Maybe I shouldn't feel so badly about it. Maybe it's a good thing
      I let my anger out. I had to do something.

Using Transference as an Aid to Working Through

In addition to its myriad of functions in clarifying dynamic factors relevant to
specific problems, transference can be an important tool for working through.
The direct experience of a wish or conflict with the therapist can aid patients in
making changes.

Case Example

Mr. I (Chapters 2, 6, and 8) typically anticipated that the therapist, like his father,
would attempt to undercut him or punish him for any assertive behavior or
progress that he made in treatment. Therefore, it was significant when a dream
identified a representation of an older man who was trying to help the patient
move forward in his life:

Mr. I: I had a dream the other night that seemed different from others.
      My car was stuck, and I couldn't figure out what was wrong with
      it. An older man was there. I didn't recognize him, but somehow
      he helped me figure out what was wrong. Then I just remember
      driving it again.
Therapist: What felt different about this dream?
Mr. I: Usually I'm just stuck and nothing happens. And usually if there's
      an older guy, I'm in trouble with him. This was unusual.
Therapist: What comes to mind about it?
Mr. I: Well, I had this idea of getting advice from this older man about
      the difficulties I've been having at the company. He's a former

mentor of mine and I've always had a positive feeling about him. I
hadn't thought about him in a while but he recently came to mind.

THERAPIST: I think the older man may symbolize both your mentor and
me. The dream suggests that you're getting more comfortable
with the notion that I will not cut you down or attack you if you
feel competitive or seek my advice. Even the idea that you can get
advice from someone else is significant, as you've rarely talked
about doing this.

MR. I: I rarely do. I recognize more often now that you're trying to help
me. Not cut me down.

Thus, the patient had a shift in representation of the therapist as someone
who would undercut his assertiveness like his father to someone helpful. The
representation of another man as more responsive to him was part of an internal
change that was affecting his behavior in various circumstances. After asking for
advice from his mentor, he reported that he was feeling anxious and asked the
therapist, "Is there any problem with getting his advice?"

THERAPIST: In what way?

MR. I: I don't know. But I believe he knows my boss. What if somehow
he lets my boss know and I get into trouble?

THERAPIST: I'm not sure exactly what you would be in trouble for.

MR. I: I think my boss would be angry because he feels he knows all the
answers. Or maybe you'll be annoyed with me because I'm seeking help from someone else instead of you.

THERAPIST: It sounds like you fear I'll be competitive like your father or
boss and believe I know all the answers. I think this suggests that
when you feel safer to push a boundary to get help or ask for a
need to be met, you think you're going to get in trouble again.

MR. I: I see what you're saying. But I'm still wary about it.

In this instance Mr. I experienced backlash, fearing he would be punished by
an authority figure for his efforts to pursue his own wishes. The therapist helped
the patient recognize how he could move between a transferential view of the
therapist as undermining him and then recognize the therapist as being supportive. This information could be used to guide an ongoing shift in the patient's self
and other representations to alleviate his fears of asserting his needs with others
more generally. In addition, the more direct expression of his wishes helped to reduce the building up of his frustration and temperamental outbursts.

Applying Overlapping Dynamics to Various Problems

The dynamics that emerge for a specific problem can often be applied to others
in the process of working through. The therapist works with the patient to iden-

tify these overlapping dynamics and clarify effective interventions. The overlap allows for a better understanding of both the dynamics themselves and the degree to which the patient has been affected by them.

As described previously, Ms. C struggled with multiple problem areas. The therapist continued to aid Ms. C in the development of her understanding of how her core dynamics applied to various problems and in her ability to identify additional strategies for managing them. Her problems included

- Anxious and depressive symptoms
- Intense sadness about her daughter's going to college
- Difficulties with assertiveness
- Feelings of inadequacy and low self-esteem, associated with social anxiety
- Marital problems

Examining Ms. C's problem list had led to an increased understanding of her dynamics and progress on several fronts. The core dynamics were found to derive from pressures the patient felt to respond to the needs of others, with a fear that any effort to assert her own wishes would potentially disrupt her relationships. This led to her anger becoming self-directed or being expressed in a passive-aggressive manner, both of which left her feeling chronically frustrated. Increased recognition and tolerance of her anger eased her anxious and depressive symptoms significantly. In addition, it reduced fears that her anger would disrupt her relationships, enabling her to more directly confront her husband's criticisms and to push forward with projects at work. Her newfound assertiveness improved her confidence, easing feelings of inadequacy and low self-esteem. Her sadness about her daughter, while present, had considerably diminished, in part due to reduced dissatisfaction with her husband and her job. She continued, however, to struggle with addressing problems with her boss and her father. The therapist continued to work with these overlapping dynamics in addressing these remaining problems, including in the transference.

> Ms. C: Well, I still haven't been able to talk to my boss about the issues at work. I'm sure you're not surprised. But I have begun to focus more on my work and I'm getting more done.
> THERAPIST: What's helped you with that?
> Ms. C: I don't know exactly. I've just felt more motivation.
> THERAPIST: Maybe just being able to express your anger at the boss in here has helped with that? We did talk about how procrastinating was an indirect expression of your frustration because you felt you couldn't address problems directly with him.
> Ms. C: That could be. I did feel some relief when we went through what I would say to him and what I felt angry about. And I decided to work on my indecisiveness. I remind myself that I'm capable and I just push forward with things. I know we've talked about how I'm fearful of being assertive and how that may have interfered with my pressing ahead with projects.

THERAPIST: That's important. It seems like you're expressing your anger more effectively rather than indirectly or attacking yourself. But directly addressing the boss is still very scary.

Ms. C: I can't escape this fear that it would lead to my getting fired. And I'm still struggling with my father too. You know he was mean to my daughter, and I had to address that with him. But my daughter wants me to say more to him about his behavior.

THERAPIST: What do you think about that?

Ms. C: I just don't think I can do that. I believe it's going to really disrupt our relationship with my father, and I don't think my daughter understands. She's been distant with him.

THERAPIST: It seems just like you described how you feel with your boss: asserting yourself would end the relationship. I believe that stems from your experience with your father, as your boss has never threatened you or implied that would be the case.

Ms. C: I know but I'm still worried about it. It's true my father wouldn't talk to me for days when he was mad at me. Sometimes I wondered whether he would talk to me again! And now I realize he's really vulnerable inside. He is so easily injured.

THERAPIST: I think we've recognized that your anger feels dangerous to you and you never learned ways to feel safe addressing problems directly. Inside you believe that it can only lead to a disruption or attack. But you've found that expressing your frustration directly, as with your husband, or even describing to me your feelings toward your boss and father, has only helped. So expressing your feelings of dissatisfaction is less damaging than you thought.

Ms. C: But I feel that you must be annoyed with me for not confronting my boss when we've talked about it so much.

THERAPIST: Can you say more about that?

Ms. C: I assume you're angry. You've worked so much with me on it. And I believe you want me to accomplish this and must be frustrated. I've been worried about even bringing it up with you.

THERAPIST: It sounds like you fear I'm going to respond angrily like your father or boss. And that it would cause some disruption with me.

Ms. C: Yes, I'm worried about that.

THERAPIST: I think it's good you raised it because I actually feel you've made a lot of progress with confronting others, and I empathize with how frightening it is for you to raise your concerns. Also, we can't guarantee how your boss would react. But I'm glad you were able to bring up your concerns with me. Maybe you're frustrated that you haven't been able to talk to him.

Ms. C: Oh yes but not at you. I do recognize you hear me out, and I see you didn't attack me when I raised this with you. So I know it's safe. But my boss and father, well that's a different story.

THERAPIST: I believe the safer you feel with your anger, the more flexible you'll be about how you express it.

The following case provides an additional example of applying core dynamics to various problems of a patient with difficulties with impulse control in the course of working through.

Case Example

Ms. FF, a 42-year-old sales representative, presented with problems with impulses to buy expensive clothes and dinners. These expenditures were causing significant financial problems, and her husband had pressured her to enter treatment. She tended to minimize these purchases and reported that she did not think about them until well after they occurred. However, she intermittently would realize the extent of her spending and experience a brief wave of guilt.

While the therapist and Ms. FF were exploring this symptom, she revealed a struggle with irritability (temper episodes) and anxiety, with worries about her husband leaving her and job loss, consistent with generalized anxiety disorder (American Psychiatric Association 2013). She described recurrent conflicts in her relationships, often based on feeling slighted by others. The therapist explored her background in an effort to identify contributors to these problems.

Problem List for Ms. FF

1. Impulse control issues (shopping, temper outbursts)
2. Generalized anxiety disorder, with irritability and anxiety (fears of abandonment)
3. Relationship problems: easily feeling slighted; recurrent fights with husband and family

Ms. FF reported a troubled family history, with her parents having increasingly intense fights beginning around age 8. At age 13 her mother moved out of the family home, taking her clothes and some of the furniture with her, leaving Ms. FF and her younger brother living with their father. In addition to dealing with the abandonment by her mother, whom she saw infrequently, Ms. FF quickly became aware that her parents' money came largely from her mother's family and that they were no longer receiving these funds. Thus, the patient dealt with both the disruption of her parents' marriage and the relationship with her mother and a reduction in lifestyle. In addition, she received little explanation from either parent about what happened in their relationship and financial situation. She subsequently learned that her mother had a boyfriend and also struggled with a drinking problem.

The therapist encouraged her to pay attention to the thoughts and emotions she experienced prior to her purchases. They were able to identify that painful feelings of deprivation, abandonment, and anger preceded her buying behavior. The therapist pointed out the connection to the traumatic events of her childhood.

> Ms. FF: So I noticed the other day that just before I went shopping I was really mad at my husband.
> THERAPIST: What happened at that time?
> Ms. FF: Well, I just became infuriated with him. He claims he's tired from working and when he gets home he just sits there and watches TV. It's like somehow I'm supposed to manage the kids and make dinner. It's like I'm all on my own.

THERAPIST: That sounds like how you felt when your mother left—abandoned, deprived, and feeling you had to manage more on your own.

Ms. FF: I guess so. I mean I did end up having to do more chores then and take care of my younger brother. My mom couldn't be bothered. Anyway, I was still mad at my husband the next day. Then I marched over to the store and bought two outfits. I felt better, but now I think I should probably return them.

THERAPIST: I think as you become more aware of your feelings you can look for other ways to express them besides shopping.

Ms. FF: Maybe. I know that on the rare occasions I saw my mom, she used to take me shopping. Those times felt really important.

The therapist and patient discussed further how purchasing items or experiences (e.g., dinners at nice restaurants) felt like a connection to her mother. However, these purchases would only briefly relieve her feelings of deprivation and frustration. As these dynamics and approaches to her shopping impulses were identified, the therapist increasingly focused on the patient's other problems, including anxiety and irritability, and conflicts with her husband and friends. She would frequently feel as if others were ignoring and dismissing her and accuse them of being mean.

Ms. FF: My husband is such an asshole. I'm just fed up with him. Recently he's been coming home late from his job, but he's not making much money. I lost my temper and was screaming at him last night.

THERAPIST: How did he respond to you?

Ms. FF: Well, he just gets mad and keeps quiet. But I'm actually really worried that maybe he's having an affair or something and he's just going to leave. I'm like worrying about it all the time!

THERAPIST: Is this a new worry?

Ms. FF: No, I've had it on and off over the years.

THERAPIST: Was there ever any evidence of an affair?

Ms. FF: No. I actually kind of doubt it. He's not really the type. He generally keeps to himself.

THERAPIST: I wonder if this is another example of you fearing you're going to be abandoned.

Ms. FF: You mean I think he'll leave me because of what happened with my mother?

THERAPIST: Yes.

Ms. FF: That could be true. Because I also worry about the same thing with my job. But I've been at this company for 20 years, and I always get positive feedback on my annual reviews!

It emerged that many of the patient's generalized anxiety symptoms were related to fears of abandonment, because she constantly felt the threat of rejection and loss. In addition, her irritability frequently was triggered by these perceived threats. When her problems with relationship conflicts were explored, she was prone to feeling abandoned, slighted, or ignored, leading to recurrent fights with her circle of friends.

> Ms. FF: So I found out that Jill and Marissa got together and never even told me about it. I saw a picture of them online! So I confronted Jill about it. She said, "I can get together with whomever I want." I told her it was nasty not to invite me. Now I'm worrying that maybe I pushed her away, but I don't even want to talk to her for a while.
>
> THERAPIST: I do think you're prone to feeling slighted. It seems you're on the lookout for other people behaving in a rejecting way or excluding you. Here again the experience with your family comes to mind, as you really felt shoved aside by your parents' problems.
>
> Ms. FF: Yeah. You know I still have these problems with my mother. In fact, I wanted to talk to her about this incident, but she didn't seem to be paying attention. It was infuriating. I think maybe she had been drinking.

Thus, the therapist and patient continued to explore how her traumatic history, self/other representations, and dynamic factors contributed to her expectations of being attacked and abandoned, leading to her shopping impulses, anxiety and irritability, and relationship conflicts. The therapist also helped the patient recognize that her attacks on others when she felt slighted added further to her stress, as she feared pushing others away. As part of the working-through process, her increased understanding of her difficulties helped her to be less reactive to perceived threats and enabled her to find more adaptive ways of handling her difficulties, such as increased communication with others about her concerns before they exploded into conflict.

References

American Psychiatric Association: Diagnostic and Statistical Manual of Mental Disorders, 5th Edition. Arlington, VA, American Psychiatric Association, 2013

Freud S: Remembering, repeating and working-through (further recommendations on the technique of psycho-analysis II) (1914), in The Standard Edition of the Complete Psychological Works of Sigmund Freud, Vol 12. Translated by Strachey J. London, Hogarth, 1958, pp 147–156

Freud S: Some character-types met with in psychoanalytic work (1916), in The Standard Edition of the Complete Psychological Works of Sigmund Freud, Vol 14. Translated by Strachey J. London, Hogarth, 1957, pp 309–333

10

Managing Termination

By identifying a set of targeted problems in problem-focused psychodynamic psychotherapy (PrFPP), therapists and patients can establish parameters by which to assess improvement in therapy (Table 10–1), a significant difference from more traditional psychodynamic psychotherapies and psychoanalysis (Gabbard 2009; Schlesinger 2013; Ticho 1972; Tyson 1996; Weinshel 1992). When considering a plan for termination, they can discuss progress toward various goals and the degree of resolution of specific problems. As in most psychodynamic psychotherapies, patients' transferential feelings and fantasies about the treatment ending, including anger and sadness, provide additional opportunities to address a variety of problems. Although therapists and patients intend for difficulties to be diminished or resolved, they may determine that changes in certain problems may be limited or not possible. In these circumstances the therapists work to improve the patient's ability to tolerate and manage these persistent issues.

To illustrate the problem-focused approach to termination, we will describe a patient who dealt with depression and anxiety, feelings of exclusion by her daughter, aging issues, and unresolved anger and guilt toward her ex-husband and mother, all of which interfered with pursuing a new intimate relationship (Tables 10–2 through 10–4). Increased self-understanding, reduced affective symptoms, an improved relationship with her daughter, and a resumption of dating were used as markers to plan treatment termination.

Case Example

Ms. GG, a 63-year-old divorced psychotherapist, presented with a down and anxious mood, low energy, poor concentration, and insomnia. She began treatment with PrFPP, and the therapist prescribed venlafaxine, with the dosage increased to 150 mg/day, which provided partial resolution of her depressive

145

TABLE 10–1.	Termination in problem-focused psychodynamic psychotherapy

Problem focus identifies parameters to evaluate progress.

Assess the degree of resolution of specific problems.

Use transference to address remaining difficulties.

Encourage tolerance and adaptation for persistent problems.

disorder. As the therapist and Ms. GG began exploring her symptoms, they identified several contextual contributors and related problem areas. She was distressed by severe back problems that visibly affected her gait and had led to her significantly cutting back on seeing patients. Her reduction in practice greatly diminished the satisfaction that she obtained from her work. Overall the patient felt marginalized and useless, believing that others were no longer interested in or needed her. In addition to missing her patients and not having an intimate relationship with a man, she focused on her daughter Amy, whom she experienced as neglectful, disinterested, and unwilling to help her now that she was getting older. She had one son, whom she viewed as less rejecting and withholding, but their relationship was limited, in part because he lived in another state.

By monitoring contexts, the therapist and Ms. GG initially identified that feelings of aloneness or exclusion triggered surges in her depressive symptoms. These feelings commonly followed conversations with her daughter in which she believed that Amy dismissed her wishes to have more contact. She was frustrated rather than empathic with her daughter's level of involvement with her husband and three teenage children. "She doesn't care about me. Maybe it's because of how she felt I treated her father in the divorce," Ms. GG would aver, despite it being evident that her daughter was friendly when they did get together.

Exploration of these problems brought to mind her relationship with her mother, in which she experienced herself as the parent attempting to soothe her mother's catastrophic preoccupations, including hypochondriacal fears. Ms. GG believed her mother lacked boundaries in demanding the patient's attention, and she felt guilty when she set limits with her mother. She had been careful to not pressure her daughter to respond to her needs and worries as her mother did with her, but then felt frustrated that Amy was not more responsive. It became clear that Ms. GG was indirectly expressing anger toward Amy related to her own mother, who was typically focused on her own concerns rather than the patient's.

When asked what communication she had had with her daughter about these problems, Ms. GG revealed that she had not talked with Amy about her frustrations, becoming preoccupied about how to best express her feelings. As the therapist explored this inhibition with her, Ms. GG acknowledged fears that expressing her anger, which was very intense, would drive Amy further away. In obtaining additional developmental history, the patient described great distress at her father's intermittent outbursts of temper, which felt uncontrolled and fright-

TABLE 10–2. **Problem list and indicators of progress for Ms. GG**

Problem	Content	Indicator of Response
Depressive and anxious symptoms	Feelings of marginalization, anger at daughter	Reduction in feelings of neglect, depression
Fear of expressing anger/ unassertiveness	Fear of discussing frustration directly with daughter	Ability to talk to daughter about her frustrations
Dependency as dangerous	Fear of expressing need for help	Ability to seek help, rather than see it as humiliating
Fear of aging	Aging as creating helplessness, dependency	Acknowledgment, tolerance of aging fears
Lack of relationships with men	Regrets about her marriage, lack of mourning of ex-husband	Renewed efforts to meet men

ening to the patient, and served to bully others to do what he wanted. She felt the urge to coerce her daughter to respond, a form of identification with the aggressor, which then led to a wave of guilty feelings. Indeed, when asked what she might say to Amy, Ms. GG responded, "I would tell her, 'I think that you don't want to get together, and you aren't concerned about me and I want to understand why.'" The therapist and she discussed the resentment evident in her proposed communication, noting the link to her father's anger. They discussed more productive ways of expressing her frustration with Amy.

> Ms. GG: I'm just so irritated with her. I feel she doesn't care about me. She just ignores me. And she has no interest in my health. I think maybe I should tell her that.
> THERAPIST: Well, I'm concerned that your daughter might hear that as an accusation and feel judged. It could get her back up.
> Ms. GG: You're probably right. What would you suggest?
> THERAPIST: Something like, "I feel you don't want to get together with me. I wonder if something's bothering you." Or, "I'd like to talk to you more about my health problems but it's difficult for me, and I'm worried you won't want to talk about them."

This type of intervention, suggesting scripts for ways of communicating, is not standard for traditional psychodynamic psychotherapy; alongside these suggestions, the therapist suggested a formulation for her difficulties:

TABLE 10–3. Dynamic formulation for Ms. GG

Self/other representations:	Self as angry; others as potentially damaged or rejecting
	Self as needy; others as intruded upon, rejecting
	Self as smothered, guilty; others as needy, demanding
Developmental contributors:	Mother displayed needy, anxious, and intrusive behavior, demanding the patient's attention. Her father was temperamental and bullying.
Conflicts and defenses:	Patient fears her angry and dependent wishes will damage others or cause rejection. Defenses include avoidance, undoing, reaction formation, and identification with the aggressor.
Interpersonal relationships:	Self/other representations and conflicts lead to dissatisfaction with relationships, including feeling a lack of responsiveness of others to her needs and wishes.

Ms. GG: Well, those are a lot better. Can I write them down?

Therapist: Sure. But I think you have difficulty controlling and managing your anger at Amy and that you see her somewhat like your mother. It's as if you feel you have to take care of her needs and not express your concerns. Then you get mad but worry it will emerge in a temper outburst like your father's.

Ms. GG: Yes, and then I would feel terrible about it. I get stuck. Maybe we can write down your suggestions. I want to go over them before I talk to her.

Therapist: I think that would be a good idea.

Although she became more comfortable expressing angry feelings in general, the patient continued to avoid having a conversation with her daughter about her concerns. This inhibition led Ms. GG to become frustrated with both herself and with her therapist. In this vignette the transference was used to address this anger as part of the working-through process.

Ms. GG: I can't seem to talk to her. I'm not sure whether that's your fault or my fault.

Therapist: I guess one aspect of what we want to understand is why is someone to blame? What's your sense of both of our roles?

Ms. GG: I see what you're saying about blaming. I tended to blame myself growing up for my parents' fights. I thought maybe I made them miserable. And I didn't have any siblings that could help.

Therapist: I think you also ended up expressing anger at them toward yourself. And what about now with us?

TABLE 10–4. Interventions for therapy with Ms. GG

Identify that anger is not necessarily damaging to others and may be expressed in a productive manner.

Help her recognize that needs are not inherently "needy" or damaging.

Help her recognize guilt related to mother in asking others for help, presuming that such requests would be damaging or intrusive as she experienced with her mother.

Help her understand that wishes for help can be expressed in an effective manner without being damaging or intrusive.

Identify how her father's behavior contributed to her fears and perception of her anger as damaging.

Help her recognize how denying her wishes results in their intensification because she is not able to obtain what she needs from others.

Increase her sense of safety in communicating these desires, leading to more responsiveness from others along with decreased feelings of marginalization.

Ms. GG: I just feel like I'm not getting it done. What's wrong with me? I should be able to say something, but I end up on the phone with her and let the conversation pass by without saying anything.

THERAPIST: I think you must really struggle because you felt you couldn't get mad at your parents and had to just look out for their moods. It must have been very scary to think about raising your frustrations with them.

Ms. GG: I don't remember having ever considered it, but I don't think that would have gone over too well.

THERAPIST: And what about with me?

Ms. GG: Well, you don't seem to be helping me get this done. It's frustrating. I know we've made progress, but I need to talk with Amy.

THERAPIST: It sounds like you're angry with me.

Ms. GG: I guess you could say that. But I know you're trying to help.

THERAPIST: It seems scary to tell me you're mad.

Ms. GG: Yes, but I feel relieved now being able to say it. I'm beginning to feel safer with expressing my wishes in general. I finally told off my friend who kept canceling our get togethers, so I know something's changing.

Addressing Fears of Revealing Needs

As discussed in Chapter 9, problems can persist because more than one dynamic factor is contributing to them. Upon further exploration of her ongoing struggles in communicating with her daughter, the therapist and Ms. GG determined that she was conflicted about revealing her needs to her children. These included wishes to get help with certain chores made difficult by her back problems. These fears were found to relate in part to conflicts deriving from problems with her mother. She described that her mother had often complained about being sick, sought the patient's attention, and thought Ms. GG's role was to calm and care for her. Ms. GG found these tasks to be highly intrusive and annoying, because she felt pressured to respond. She stated, "I never wanted to expose my children to that." The therapist and patient determined that Ms. GG equated any requests for help from her children to her mother's demanding and controlling behavior, inhibiting her efforts to seek support from them.

> THERAPIST: You've always presented yourself as very independent because you did not want your children to experience what you did with your mother. Now you want more support from Amy, but you're in conflict about it. You really haven't told her you need help, and she's not used to responding to you in this way. We need to understand more about your fears of being vulnerable, and figure out how to develop a language to communicate what help you need.
>
> Ms. GG: I guess I really don't want to ask for help. I want to think of myself as super-independent. I don't want to see myself as being like my mother. She was just constantly pressing me with her worries about everything. I had to put up a wall to protect myself.
>
> THERAPIST: I believe you view any request for help as being exactly like your mother, even though you rarely make such requests. So I think you've compensated with this hyper-independence and don't allow yourself to ask for any support.
>
> Ms. GG: I hadn't really considered it that way. I just like to think of myself as tough. But I guess with getting older and these back problems I really have to accept my need for help and recognize this brings up a lot of conflict for me.

After significant work on both her anger and wishes for caretaking and fears of expressing them, Ms. GG was able to talk to Amy about her dismissive behavior and believed she made some progress in getting across her concerns.

> Ms. GG: I told her that she and I were stuck in this pattern, and I wanted to try to find a way out of it. I accepted part of the blame and that I got frustrated about the limits she set.
>
> THERAPIST: That seems like a good way of saying it. So how did that go?
>
> Ms. GG: She was much more responsive than I expected. It went very well after that. I talked some about my medical problems and she seemed willing to listen. I'm worried about whether it will continue. She still doesn't have much interest in discussing our relationship.
>
> THERAPIST: I think we need to continue to examine frustrations with her as they arise, and going forward we can recall how you handled it differently this time.
>
> Ms. GG: Also, you can remind me about how much I'm still affected by my mother? I didn't realize that those problems I had with her still had so much impact.

THERAPIST: I agree we need to continue to sort through your anger and guilt about her.

Ms. GG: I think I have a pretty good idea of the things that are bothering me, but I need to find a way to keep them in mind more.

Her daughter became somewhat more solicitous, though the patient continued to be intermittently frustrated with the limits she set. She worked to accept her daughter's lack of interest in discussing their relationship, something which she very much wanted to do. She also recognized that when she was by herself for too long of a stretch, it would trigger catastrophic fears of aloneness and a low mood. She realized how her feelings were triggered not only by Amy's behavior but also by the isolation she felt in reducing her practice workload and not having a romantic partner. She arranged more regular meetings with friends and signed up for some courses, which further diminished her lonely feelings.

Exploring the Impact of Lack of an Intimate Partner

Ms. GG did not initially view the lack of an intimate relationship with a man as a problem, but she and the therapist increasingly recognized this absence contributed to her sense of aloneness and marginalization. She expressed frustration about getting together with mainly couples and feeling "like a third wheel." On exploration she revealed she had not been involved with a man in a long-term relationship since her divorce several years prior. When asked about what held her back from meeting men, she described being highly disillusioned about her marriage. She had been furious at her ex-husband for his self-focus and lack of empathy with her. She felt that her interest in another relationship had been dampened by years of bullying and feeling misunderstood.

Shortly after beginning treatment, her ex-husband died unexpectedly, and she was surprised at how much it affected her. She felt a surge of grief, remembering how she felt he rescued her from her family and positive experiences they had shared early in their marriage and with the children. This period of sadness was followed by a wave of guilt about hurtful things she believed she had done to him. For example, she felt guilty about having "kicked him out," because he had not wanted the divorce. After realizing the struggles she had with her daughter, she became aware that she had not assertively expressed her needs and frustrations with him. She wondered if he would have responded differently had she been clearer.

The therapist continued to work with her in the mourning process. He empathized with Ms. GG but indicated that there were good reasons she split up with him, which she had described previously, and she was brushing aside those problems in the wake of his death. Indeed, her guilt was followed by a resurgence of anger at what she viewed as his arrogance and lack of response to her frustrations. Her rage eventually subsided, after which she experienced a recurrence of sadness about the loss of the positive aspects of their relationship, including the feeling that he had rescued her from her family. After a couple months her preoccupation with him subsided, and she began to have thoughts about returning to dating. Inadequate mourning of the loss of her marriage appeared to have contributed to her avoidance of meeting men, because she had not worked through her hurt, pain, guilt, and anger. She developed a wish for a new relationship and was surprised to find herself having a "crush" on a man she met in one of her classes.

Addressing Fears About Aging

Ms. GG's back problems, which had been diagnosed as spinal stenosis, triggered worries about aging. Over time she and the therapist identified that she was anxious about becoming more dependent on her children as she aged. Additionally, she feared that her children would reject her, just as she had pushed back on her mother's needy behavior and demands for attention. Indeed, when her mother was older, Ms. GG rarely visited her, because she anticipated being overwhelmed by her mother's demands, and she felt guilty about this. She equated dependency with both a damaging intrusiveness with others and a sense of helplessness, which was found to be a feared identification with her mother. In part because of her work on her fears of being dependent, Ms. GG came to recognize that her back problems and getting older did not mean she was helpless. She could seek help from others in a way that was not desperate or demanding. With this progress she was able to engage a part time aide.

> Ms. GG: I'm really worried about becoming helpless as I get older. I don't want to be a mess like my mother. I've just never asked for help.
> THERAPIST: I think it's important to consider that asking for help does not make you "helpless," demanding, or intrusive like your mother.
> Ms. GG: I do recognize that more, but it's still scary to feel like you can't manage on your own. However, I did contact a service to get some help. I'm going to have a woman come for a few hours twice a week.
> THERAPIST: I think that's a positive step.

Working With the Transference

As Ms. GG's improvement in a number of problem areas continued, the therapist and she discussed terminating the treatment. As noted earlier in this chapter, termination in PrFPP attends to the expression of the patient's feelings in the transference. Where possible, identifying these reactions can help further the gains in addressing particular problems. Ms. GG expressed sadness about the end of the therapeutic relationship alongside fears of managing on her own.

Ms. GG: I know from my own work with patients that it can be hard to confront the end of a relationship like this. But I've never really experienced these feelings so strongly myself. This has been really important to me. I know I can handle things on my own, but it may be sad and a bit scary managing without you. I'm worried about feeling alone and excluded again.

THERAPIST: I certainly understand those feelings. I think you're mourning the end of our relationship.

Ms. GG: What if I lose the new things I've learned?

THERAPIST: I think we should understand more about these fears of helplessness on your own. But it's also important to recognize how much you've changed. You've increased your contacts and involvement with others and addressed problems with your daughter that were triggers of depression before. And you've started dating!

Ms. GG: And here I've always made such a big deal about being independent! So I guess it's good I can acknowledge how much you've helped me and that I'll miss you.

THERAPIST: I agree. I think the idea of needing help from me was pretty scary at first.

Ms. GG: Yes, and now I recognize that and realize if I need help I'll just call you.

Encouraging Adaptation and Tolerance for Persistent Problems

The therapist and patient discussed progress thus far in terms of issues that had been dealt with and the formulation for understanding them. They also worked on accepting certain regrets in her life.

Ms. GG: So where are we in this? I think I'm doing very well. You've really helped me tremendously. I like how you work in therapy by addressing specific problems.

THERAPIST: I think you've really moved forward in dealing with your difficulties, and it has been a very positive and productive relationship.

Ms. GG: I still kind of doubt I'll be able to find a new boyfriend, but I've enjoyed getting out more. I feel less lonely. But I do regret that I didn't run my life differently. I should have recognized the problems with my husband. I knew something was wrong.

THERAPIST: It's easy to retrospectively judge how one could have done better. You said that when you married him that wives were expected to follow what their husbands told them to do. Things have changed since then. And you also said how he rescued you from your family.

Ms. GG: That's true about social mores changing. When I decided to get divorced from him nobody supported me. They all thought I should stay with him.

The therapist acknowledged the difficulties that being a woman created in trying to address problems with her husband. Ms. GG was able to reveal and work with her frustrations about termination in the setting of a discussion about an end date for therapy.

THERAPIST: Why don't we talk about setting a date for stopping?

Ms. GG: I guess that's a good idea. Of course I'm still frustrated about the way certain things are in my life, like my back problems and the issues with my daughter.

THERAPIST: Do you feel frustrated with me?

Ms. GG: I guess in a way. I wish you could have helped me get closer to my daughter and get a boyfriend. But I realize from my own work that a therapist can't produce miracles.

THERAPIST: I agree with you, but it's also good that you can readily express frustration with me. We also know you've been able to accept or at least tolerate certain problems in your life. And you've taken steps to deal with these issues, including getting help at home, arranging more activities, and even going on some dates. Maybe you'll be able to make further progress in these areas.

Ms. GG: Yeah, I kind of doubt things will change much. But you're absolutely right that I have more skills for dealing with these issues. Now I recognize early on if there's a problem. What do you think about me checking in with you in 6 months?

THERAPIST: Sure, that sounds good.

As alluded to above, Ms. GG, who had been in two prior psychotherapeutic treatments, found PrFPP to be particularly helpful. She averred that the problem-focused approach provided a framework for using her insight to better address the difficulties she was facing. When the patient checked in with the therapist 6 months after termination, it became apparent that the skills she developed helped her to independently manage ongoing problems in her life.

References

Gabbard GO: What is a "good enough" termination? J Am Psychoanal Assoc 57(3):575–594, 2009 19620466

Schlesinger HJ: Endings and Beginnings: On Terminating Psychotherapy and Psychoanalysis. New York: Routledge, 2013.

Ticho EA: Termination of psychoanalysis: treatment goals, life goals. Psychoanal Q 41(3):315–333, 1972 5047036

Tyson P: Termination of psychoanalysis and psychotherapy, in Textbook of Psychoanalysis. Edited by Nersessian E, Kopff RG Jr. Washington, DC, American Psychiatric Press, 1996, pp 501–524

Weinshel EM: Therapeutic technique in psychoanalysis and psychoanalytic psychotherapy. J Am Psychoanal Assoc 40(2):327–347, 1992 1593075

Index